RT34 .P38 2013
Patrick, William B
The call of nursing

S0-DFG-437

DISCARDED

Colorado Mountain College
Quigley Library
3000 County Road 114
Glenwood Springs, CO
81601

The CALL of NURSING

The CALL of NURSING

Voices from the Front Lines of Health Care

WILLIAM B. PATRICK

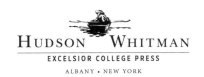

HUDSON WHITMAN

EXCELSIOR COLLEGE PRESS

ALBANY • NEW YORK

Copyright 2013 by
Hudson Whitman/ Excelsior College
All rights reserved.
No part of this book may be reproduced or transmitted in any form
or by any means, electronic or mechanical, including photocopying,
recording, or by any information storage and retrieval system,
without permission in writing from the publisher.

All material has been used with the permission of the participants.

Published in the United States by
Hudson Whitman/ Excelsior College Press
7 Columbia Circle, Albany, NY 12203
www.hudsonwhitman.com

Printed in the United States of America
Book design by Melissa Mykal Batalin
Cover design by Phil Pascuzzo

Library of Congress
Cataloging-in-publication data
LCCN: 2013933927
ISBN: 978-0-9768813-6-0 (hardcover)
ISBN: 978-0-9768813-7-7 (paperback)

Thus in silence in dreams' projections,

Returning, resuming, I thread my way through the hospitals,

The hurt and wounded I pacify with soothing hand,

I sit by the restless all the dark night, some are so young,

Some suffer so much, I recall the experience sweet and sad....

—Excerpt from "The Wound-Dresser" by Walt Whitman

CONTENTS

FOREWORD

Occupational stories can serve as powerful tools: they can educate us about the details of a specific job, illustrate various realities within that career, and enrich our emotional and spiritual lives, all at the same time. The compelling narratives in *The Call of Nursing: Voices from the Front Lines of Health Care* certainly fulfill all those expectations. While treating us like trusted confidantes, these nurses allow us to peek behind the curtain of a profession that deals with individuals at their most vulnerable times – when they are patients.

These twenty-three, first-person profiles in nursing are ethnically, culturally, and educationally diverse. Some of the women and men here emulated mothers who were nurses, and were sure of their life paths before they entered high school. Some switched careers in midstream, for better salaries or increased job security, among other things. And others came to nursing much later in life, often answering a mysterious call to follow a vocation that could make a difference for individuals in need. But, taken together, their stories chronicle work experiences and environments that not only illuminate the broad range of career options for nurses but also form a valuable body of health care knowledge. All in all, this book communicates the essence of nursing.

The profound qualities that unite the voices we hear in this book are passion for the profession and compassion for patients. Whether you read this book from cover to cover or savor these nurses' lives one at a time, you can't help but be moved by their hopes, their struggles, and their joys. If you are a nurse, you'll recognize yourself somewhere in here. If you're lucky enough to have a nurse as a friend or family member, you will probably rush through reading it so you can share these stories with them. And if you aren't a nurse yet, I guarantee this book will make you consider becoming one.

Gertrude B. Hutchinson, MSIS, MA, RN, CCRN-R
Archivist, Bellevue Alumnae Center for Nursing History

The CALL of NURSING

DR. COLLEEN WALSH

I have worked as a nurse on orthopedic units at Level I trauma centers in Boston, in Albany, New York, in Charlottesville, Virginia, and in Ann Arbor, Michigan, among other places, for over thirty years. I have also completed four nursing degrees while I was working full time and raising a family. In 2011, I earned my doctorate of nursing practice from the University of Southern Indiana, in Evansville, where I am currently an assistant professor of nursing.

I always knew I was going to be a nurse. There was never a time during my early schooling, elementary through high school, when I didn't want to be one. There were absolutely no medical people in my family, so I don't know where my inspiration came from. It was just something I innately felt I wanted to do, and I never wavered from that course. I guess I was born that way.

However, I was also born with knock knees. Knock knees are when your knees rub together but your feet point out. It's the opposite of bowlegged. To make it worse, I was your typical chubby kid, and weight exacerbates that problem. My kneecaps would dislocate and at times it was very painful to walk. I had my first cast on when I was seven, and I went through my first major procedure in 1963, when I was only eleven. Over the course of my lifetime, I have undergone seven more surgical procedures to correct the problem. So I possessed a natural affinity for orthopedics because I knew what it was like to be on the other side of the cast.

When I was sixteen, after my second major procedure, a Nurse Ratched type took care of me. She made me cry every single day I was in the hospital. Now that I look back on it, though, she was probably doing what she was supposed to do. But it was the manner in which she did it. She was mean. She made fun of me and called me a baby. Even with that, I still wanted to join the profession, and I swore I would do everything I could to become the antithesis of that nurse.

On my first orthopedic rotation during nursing school, I immediately empathized with the patients. I understood the sheer magnitude of being stuck in that bed. I had experienced some of the mechanics of orthopedics, in terms of traction and weights and how they kept bones in place, and that certainly helped. I definitely knew what it felt like having little plaster crumbs under my butt, and getting a rash that drove me crazy, and how much it meant to have clean sheets. Those small things might sound unimportant, but they're magnified into an incessant form of daily torture when you're a patient.

There weren't too many of us who specialized in orthopedics when I started working. As an orthopedic nurse, I was dedicated to alleviating pain and restoring function due to musculoskeletal injuries or disorders – anything related to a bone or a joint. I have taken care of the full spectrum, from someone with a simple broken finger to someone who was completely paralyzed and on a ventilator for five years. I also treated many people, whom we called multiple-trauma patients, who suffered a combination of fractures, chest injuries, and internal injuries. Usually the other injuries healed faster than the orthopedic ones. After they passed the crisis phase in the ICU, they would come to us. I had patients who rode motorcycles and hit guardrails and left part of their shinbones behind. Their shinbones hit so hard that they just splintered into pieces and we would have to rebuild them. That was a common injury.

Orthopedic practice is very different now. We have procedures and materials we didn't have back then. We can insert artificial bone, or move bone from another part of the patient's body to fill a defect. But back in the seventies and eighties, patients with severe orthopedic injuries stayed in the hospital for months. Then, more often than not, we would see them back many times over the course of several years because of complications from the original injury. In the early days, I got to know my patients pretty well.

Now we have new orthopedic pins and rods that can actually immobilize a fracture so well that patients don't have to stay in a hospital for three or four months. They can go home in three or four days. The titanium rods we put in essentially do the job of the bone until it can heal naturally. Biologically, titanium is an inert compound, so it doesn't cause allergic reactions and isn't perceived by the body as a transplant. But normally these things are ultra-sterile. Unless there's an infection present, patients tolerate them very well. If the titanium doesn't bother a patient, we just leave it in there.

For my entire bedside career, I was fortunate enough to have worked exclusively at level I trauma centers where the sickest of the sick are found. I had exposure, every single day, to the most complex orthopedic injuries. I particularly remember one patient in Charlottesville, Virginia, in 1983. He was a twenty-five-year-old African American male who was working under his car when the blocks slipped. The engine shaft fell on his neck and severed his spinal cord at a point just below his brain. Luckily, he was close to a hospital when it happened, so he got immediate care and was placed on a ventilator. Back then, there was absolutely no nursing home or facility in the Commonwealth of Virginia that would take a patient on a ventilator. We couldn't transfer him anywhere, and he remained on my floor for five years.

From day one, we knew his condition was static – that he would always remain the way he was. He was completely paralyzed from the neck down. He couldn't breathe on his own. He couldn't speak. He only had about one square inch of skin on his neck where he could still feel any sensation at all. He was totally dependent, under our care 24/7, and the key factor in nursing him was anticipation. If, for instance, he was sitting in a chair for an hour, he couldn't feel that his butt was getting numb and pressure was building on his skin. We had to anticipate that and change his position. One of the things that we took pride in as nurses was that, for five years, this totally paralyzed man never once suffered from a bedsore.

I had been promoted to clinical head nurse on that ward and I was in charge of orienting all the new nurses. Every spring I would walk into that patient's room and say, "Listen, Phil, I've got five newbies coming this summer. Do you mind if I let them take care of you to learn how a ventilator works?" He would just look at me and cluck, and that was his okay. He was so agreeable. I trained a legion of nurses on how to manage a patient like him. I also felt it was important to recognize him as a person who still possessed a measure of autonomy – that there was nothing wrong with his head, and that he could still make decisions.

After five years, he was actually transferred to a state facility in the Virginia Beach area, and he lived another four years there. Unfortunately, he suffered an acute episode of high blood pressure that caused a cerebral hemorrhage and he died. Now I can remember dozens of patients and very specific scenarios at different hospitals. I can even recall specific room numbers for certain patients. But to this day, Phil sticks in my mind as special.

My husband and I were still living in Charlottesville when I had our first child in 1985. I had been an orthopedic nurse for thirteen years at that point, and I loved my work, but I wanted some options in my career. I wanted to be able to walk into a good hospital and say I was qualified for a high-level clinical nursing job, Monday through Friday, with no work on weekends or holidays. So I went back to school. I found that studying independently was ideal for me, and I also discovered that I was good at distance education because I was focused and self-directed. I finished all of the requirements for my bachelor's degree in April of 1988, but I couldn't attend graduation because I had just given birth to our second child.

My husband was a surgeon, and he had received a cardiothoracic surgery fellowship at the University of Michigan. He was scheduled to start that in 1989, and we moved from Charlottesville to Ann Arbor that year. With my new BSN in hand, I really did walk in and say that I wanted a clinical nurse job, Monday through Friday. Well, the Chairman of Orthopedics in Virginia knew the Chairman of Orthopedics in Ann Arbor, and they conspired to help me. I was the first nurse who ever held a jointly funded appointment. I only had to work a Christmas holiday once, and I was on call just one weekend every six months.

When I was Clinical Care Coordinator in Trauma/Orthopedics at the University of Michigan Medical Center, we had a remarkable patient. I ended up publishing an article about him in a nursing journal and identified him by a pseudonym – Mr. Michael. He was sixty-three years old, with a twenty-year history of rheumatoid arthritis, and he was admitted with a debilitating neck deformity and venous stasis ulcers. Over the course of time, his neck had become so deformed that his right ear literally sat on his shoulder. We could lift his head about two inches, but he demonstrated no active cervical motion, and the change had occurred so gradually that his eyes had actually adjusted. If I had put my ear on my right shoulder, I would have been looking sideways. Mr. Michael's eyes had moved so that, even with a cervical spine deformity clinically measuring ninety degrees, he was looking straight at us. That was a little unnerving, to say the least.

He obviously had a lot of problems swallowing, eating, and breathing, so we evaluated him to help straighten out his neck. If we could somehow reposition it and fuse it in that new position, it could heal that way. But straightening it wasn't so simple. What we had to do was put him in traction, with pulleys on his head, and the traction pulled only in one direction. His muscles had gotten used to being in that position. Every couple of days, we would change the traction. We could only move it maybe an inch at a time, because those tight muscles had to adjust to each new position.

My job was to coordinate all the care he got. Every day I would perform a specific assessment to make sure all of the nerves were still functional. If everything was progressing smoothly, I would adjust the traction. If he had a problem, I was the one who called the orthopedist. We had to go gradually, over the course of several weeks, and we had to make sure that his eyes readjusted during that time.

We did a lot of preplanning and we anticipated a diverse range of potential problems. We had multiple medical services evaluate him prior to surgery, because if we didn't have a chance to be successful, then it really would have been a disservice to put Mr. Michael through all of that. The surgery was the very last and essentially the easiest of the entire process, and the surgeon who operated on him was excellent. Mr. Michael stayed in the hospital about ten weeks and was discharged with his neck completely straight and his eyes pointed in the right direction.

That was an important case for me because it was one where all the doctors respected my knowledge and were confident of my abilities to manage a delicate situation. At the time, I was able to function more as a nurse practitioner than as a nurse, and that experience led me to another career change. I just felt that I had gotten to a point where I needed a new challenge.

We moved to Mobile, Alabama, in 1991 when my husband got a faculty position there, and I went to graduate school. I got a master's degree as a Clinical Nurse Specialist in 1993, and then a year after that, I decided I wanted to be a nurse practitioner. I knew I didn't want to do just snotty noses and ear infections, so I went into a post-master's acute care nurse practitioner program. That was a program geared toward nurses working with specialties in a hospital setting. That concept drew on the skill set that I had acquired by working in big hospitals and taking care of really sick patients. I finished in November of 1995 and took the first national certification exam.

In most states, nurse practitioners have to practice in collaboration with physicians. There are some things that we can't do, of course, because we don't have the training. For example, we can't do surgeries. We can certainly recognize major problems that are in need of a higher level of care than we can provide, and that's why most states have laws stipulating that nurse practitioners must enter into a collaborative practice agreement with a physician. We couldn't get hospital privileges to work in a hospital and see patients if we didn't have those agreements.

But I believe that, as a nurse practitioner, I can offer something holistic that many doctors don't provide: I view my patients from a different perspective. I'm able to look at not just the disease but the patient with the disease. I carefully consider patients' responses to therapies that we've ordered. I assess them for changes and decide if I need to alter our orders. I write orders; I don't take orders. That's a big difference. I don't want to generalize but, again, nurses and nurse practitioners tend to look at patients in a different way. It isn't necessarily a good or a bad thing – it's just the nature of our education. Nurses bring something different to the table.

When you've been a nurse at the bedside in major teaching hospitals for as long as I have, you've seen literally thousands of patients over the course of your career. I couldn't help but become emotionally involved with many of them. Actually, if I saw someone who didn't get involved, I wondered about that person as a nurse. And it was inevitable that I carried some of those emotions home with me. That happened a lot when I was young but, as I got older, I was able to put things in a little bit more perspective. I learned, for self-preservation, to compartmentalize: *This is happening at work and needs to stay here; now I've left work, and this is what I care about at home.* I can't explain, step by step, how you compartmentalize horrible trauma. It's not something that I consciously did. I think it was in part a learned skill, and probably part defense mechanism, but it was a necessary component of the job. Working as a nurse practitioner moved me even a little further from that emotional involvement with my patients, and it was probably my first step toward realizing that I wanted to broaden my ability to help people.

I remember, when I first contemplated becoming a teacher, that I was really concerned about leaving the bedside. One of my mentors said to me, "Well, if you take care of the patient at the bedside, then you can change the life of that one person. But if you teach dozens of nurses to change a life at the bedside, you've increased what you're able to accomplish." And I realized that, even as a nurse practitioner, I found that patients didn't understand what I was talking about much of the time. They suffered from a medical problem and they had come to me to fix that problem, but I seldom had the opportunity to have a complex and stimulating medical discussion with them.

So now I work as a full-time assistant professor of nursing at the University of Southern Indiana in Evansville, Indiana, and I love it. I teach online, which I think is the funny part of this entire process. I earned my bachelor's degree as a distance education student and all of my teaching is now online. As an educator, I definitely have to be far more global and knowledgeable about a lot of different things. I do miss the hands-on nursing, although I do go around and see patients with my students when they're getting their clinical experiences.

Each aspect of nursing, each separate part of nursing, offers a different kind of satisfaction. I can't make a hierarchy out of them. Being a nurse isn't easy. You sure don't get paid real well. But it is a profession that can allow you to achieve potentials you didn't realize you could reach. I grew up in a very blue-collar family and my parents said that the only way to become a nurse was to go to a hospital to learn. They told me you didn't go to college to become a nurse. That's how I ended up in a three-year diploma program. I went to the school of nursing at Massachusetts General Hospital because that was what was available to me at the time. I was just a kid who went off to a three-year hospital program, but at least that became the springboard for everything else. There are so many more options now. As I tell my students, you're never too old to learn. And you shouldn't believe you're ever too old to achieve what you want, either.

BLYTHE HARRISON-SAYRE

I worked for almost thirty years at the same hospital in Portland, Oregon, and married a fellow respiratory therapist. We had one child and then adopted four, two from Russia and two from Kazakhstan. The kids' needs were many and varied, and going back to school seemed impossible until 2008.

I was involved in a situation with a patient who developed malignant ascites, which is a fluid collection in the abdomen. The fluid had shifted out of his intravascular system, caused a collapse, and he had arrested. They had resuscitated him, and then brought him down to our ICU. At the shift change, when I walked in, a resident and an intern were putting in central IV lines – large-bore IV catheters. "You know this patient's pH level was below survivability and you guys did not treat," I said.

"We're busy putting in lines here," the resident answered.

"Okay, well, I think we need to do an arterial blood gas test, and I think we need to do some more treating."

He looked over and said, "You know you're just the RT, right?"

Right. I was only the respiratory therapist. My knee-jerk reaction was to think, *Listen, buddy, my level of knowledge about respiratory and blood gases you can't even begin to touch.* I knew, of course, that would be the wrong response. But then I thought, *I have this knowledge.* We can work with it, and we can help this patient. It's not about the lines. It's about the patient. Putting in lines was an important part of what was going on, but it wasn't the whole focus. Getting the homeostasis back was a significant part of it, too.

Within fifteen minutes, we had another code on our hands, and the patient didn't survive. I can't know, given the patient's age and all the other co-morbidities, if he would have survived had they listened to me. But to be told I was only the RT, that I didn't really have solid input there, and to be quiet? That really rubbed me the wrong way, and it was the final straw. I had been practicing respiratory therapy for a long time, and I could do it with my eyes closed and my hands tied behind my back, half asleep, and do it really well, but that didn't seem to matter. At that moment, I knew I needed to go somewhere else.

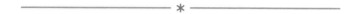

After thirty years in the health care field, I felt like I had to work a little faster, a little harder, to prove the old, gray synapses inside my head were still firing efficiently. A coworker at the hospital had encouraged me to look at a "distance" nursing program, but I was uncertain about whether I could make the leap to online learning. My educational history had always included the typical classroom scenario with an instructor and me taking notes by hand – nothing with a computer – so I wasn't sure I could master all the new technology. To be honest, at the start, copy and paste were monumental events in my day. So the change involved a huge learning curve for me, but it worked. I passed all my courses without any problems.

I formed a study group for the capstone examination with seven other students in the Portland area. We met once a week, testing and checking each others' skills, collaborating on the best ways to study, Skyping with students in Tennessee and Wyoming, and always cheering each other on. I graduated in September of 2010. As a graduation present to myself, I boarded a plane to Peru, volunteering with the medical mission group, CardioStart International, the very same day.

CardioStart's humanitarian missions provide free heart surgery and medical services to children and adults in developing countries. They go everywhere, from Vietnam to Uganda to Peru. I am fluent in Spanish, and they don't have respiratory therapists in Peru, so I went along as an RT and an RN and a translator. I was one member of the team of thirty-five cardiologists, cardiac surgeons, and ICU nurses who went there. Our lead surgeon, Dr. Mariano Brizzio, was born in Argentina but works out of New Jersey.

Saturday, Sept. 17 – Arrived in Peru very early morning, though it felt like two days later after 26 hours in planes and layovers. Something very different in the air – less oxygen. Only about 19% at this altitude, and you know it just walking around. So out to the market for water and breakfast munchies. Generally working out the soreness from so many hours in the planes. Very noticeable – I'm at least a foot and a half taller than everyone else! Traffic is breathtaking – jump back & suck air 'cause they will run right over you. Horns honking, but no cursing. Spanish is rapidly coming back – wish I could tune out some of the comments.

That's part of my first journal entry from the trip. We were in Arequipa, Peru's second-largest city, with almost 850,000 people, surrounded by snow-capped volcanoes. They have no MRIs, no CT scans, and no Peruvian cardiac surgery team operating there. It's an awfully big city not to have a cardiovascular team. So anybody who needed life-saving heart surgery had to travel about 800 miles to the capital, Lima. For the patients who are selected for the free surgeries provided by CardioStart, it's almost like winning the lottery of life because, for all practical purposes, there's no other way they could get the critical care they need there.

But getting anything done in Peru was often difficult, and corruption was incessant. The Peruvian government inspectors even demanded a bribe to release our shipping container of donated medical supplies. "If you want your container, you're going to have to pay $10,000 U.S.," they told us. "Wait a minute," our doctors said. "These are all donated supplies that we're giving to the Peruvian hospital for your people. Why would you charge us?" No amount of logic or reason would work. Bribery is what greases the wheels down there.

Sunday, Sept. 18 – Everyone is up early and very excited. The national security police and hospital assistants arrived in the hospital's best ambulance and 1959 Chevrolet Apache truck to take all of us and the bags of donated supplies to the hospital. There are 70 large luggage bags of donated equipment. This is a large, 6-floor hospital building that is all glass windows and concrete. Inside is quite a shock for the 20 team members who weren't here last year. Think 1950-1960 with paint peeling on the concrete walls – old institution green still reigns as the supreme color choice. Old metal bar gurneys (no pads), oxygen tanks (H size which are taller than Amber) standing all over the place. These are 6-8 bed units without even any curtains between beds. The absolute barest minimum of anything anywhere.

CardioStart goes to Peru the same three weeks every year, and families wait all year for them, watching for the announcement on the front page of the daily newspapers. The hospital itself plays it up because it's definitely a huge service that they wouldn't have without CardioStart. It's a big production. The Peruvian system is very different from our medical system. Almost nobody has insurance there, so they really have to be proactive for themselves and their families.

When we arrived, our team held an open cardiovascular clinic to assess the potential patients and see which ones might be the most likely candidates for successful surgery. Many people sat for hours, waiting to be seen. Our team brought a state-of-the-art ultrasound machine and an ultrasound technician who worked with the cardiologists to help them diagnose the various congenital heart defects. Often, with congenital heart abnormalities, people won't have enough oxygen in their systems, and they literally become very cachectic – thin and frail – because they can't eat. They don't even have enough oxygen reserve to spend the time eating – they're just too tired. They become physically disabled and unable to participate in surgery. And their physical presentation at that clinic was more than significant: it became a functional death sentence for several patients who were just too sick to survive the surgery. Our doctors had to review all of the histories and decide who could have surgery and who couldn't, literally making life-changing decisions. What a terrible responsibility. "You can have surgery. You can't."

Tuesday, Sept. 20 – Our adult patient today is a young lady of 25 who has to make a very important decision. There is no tissue aortic valve here to fit her, and if we do surgery, she will have to get a mechanical valve and will have to avoid having any more kids. She has one daughter. Then she will also have to be on blood thinners, as well as facing possible valve replacement later in life (if even possible here). She tells Dr. Brizzio that she can't even play or run with her 3-year-old. Her decision is to have surgery so she can "be a total mom and wife." The husband supports her (very unusual in this macho society where having a son is a big issue) and obviously adores her.

Knowing Spanish and acting as translator made my job much easier. They could send me up or down the stairs, and I could find my way everywhere. They could send me to check on the patients, and I could communicate easily with them. I could provide not only the pre-op teaching before the open heart surgery, but I could also reinforce a lot of the post-op training. The families usually take care of the surgical patients there, and they don't let them lift a finger, which is counterproductive. We wanted them up. We wanted them moving. We wanted them coughing and deep breathing and taking care of themselves, with very few exceptions. We certainly didn't want them lifting anything heavy or pushing with their arms, but we wanted them to be as active as possible afterwards because rheumatic fever is still common in Peru and that causes damage to mitral valves.

Lungs are dark and moist and wet, and if you get any kind of a bug that wants to start a pneumonia, those lungs make secretions every day, and you have to keep coughing and coughing. That hurts a lot after you've had your chest split open, and your natural tendency is to avoid doing it. That's one of the reasons why I teach pre-operatively. I tell my patients, "This is what you should expect. This is how you're going to cough. This is what you're going to do to help your lungs, and this is why you're going to do it." If they listen and learn, they'll have a much better chance of avoiding infections and surviving. Hearing instructions for the first time through post-operative pain, within a fog of medications, perhaps scared of all of the strange people around you, makes assimilating that important information quite a bit harder.

I brought a lot of respiratory equipment down to Peru. I had purchased pulse oximeter probes to record the patient's oxygen levels, and I went out to the mercado and bought the little clay whistles that they have down there. When patients blew into the clay whistles, it would make them cough, and that's how they could get the secretions out of their lungs. It's the same for adults as it is for kids – anything you can think of to make them take a deep breath and blow. You just have to find that comfort zone with enough pain medication so they can cough, and find a device that will help them do it. I don't want to downplay the cardiac stabilization, the incredible suturing job that the docs do, and the nurses managing the medications that alter blood pressure but, post-op, getting those secretions out and getting their lungs cleared is an essential facet of recovery.

> **Sunday, Sept. 25** – *Morning and evening I go looking for all our patients to double-check how everyone's doing. Everybody coughs and deep breathes for me. I'm also double-checking all chest incisions, redoing the dressings, cutting pacer wires on the third-day post-op, giving discharge information. For me, this is just the best part, seeing them get better and making sure they have enough information to care for themselves. The families are so involved and caring. My heart is touched to see how grateful they are for our attention. I'm working very hard to be sure I follow through on everything so no one feels they didn't get what they needed.*

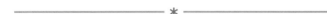

Back home in Oregon, I worked for six months in my first full-time RN position at the Oregon State Hospital, which is a chronic psych facility for civilly committed patients. "Civilly committed" means that there was nothing of a criminal nature that got them involved with the mental health system. Part of the reason I gravitated toward the psych realm was because I wanted a strong change from my earlier work as a respiratory therapist. There, my patients were often intubated, frequently sedated, or for some other reason unable to communicate. Some of them were extremely ill for long periods of time.

The psych population I worked with was just the opposite. They were very verbal, quite active, and often confrontational. As a nurse, I had to follow a whole different set of guidelines. Just saying, "Good morning," and observing the patients' reactions, I had to assess them in a way that was clearly different than one I would use in an ICU setting. I would have to think, *Is she dressed? Is her hair brushed? Does she have eye makeup on?* Even small details like that would offer important indications about a patient's mental state.

However, the chronic care in that state hospital would have driven even sane people over the edge. Although most staff members were doing the best they could, the status quo there still compromised normal standards of cleanliness and safety. You couldn't even leave the hand-washing devices out because they were alcohol-based. Patients would steal them to make alcoholic drinks. The stress was much greater, in some ways, than I had ever felt working as a respiratory therapist. I put a lot of physical energy into being available in the unit, cooperating with the other nurses, and providing patient care, of course. But I also expended a lot of mental energy just trying to make little interactions positive so I could walk away feeling as if I had made some substantial difference for each patient.

But the day-to-day pressure of dealing with the verbal abuse and the physical intimidation just wore me down. I've never been called that many names by patients in such a short a period of time. And there was a patient who hit a staff member, and nothing happened to him. Then, three days later, he turned around and hit another one. When the staff member asked why, the patient said, "Because I knew you couldn't do anything about it." It was just mind-boggling.

Throwing things occurred frequently. I saw a hospital glucometer, which costs several hundred dollars and is used for testing diabetics, hurled at a nurse's head. On the particular floor where I worked, there were twenty-two nurse hires over the course of one year, and only five of us lasted more than six months.

Finally, I managed to find a job at a private hospital that incorporates acute psych, chemo dependency, and withdrawal. I work on what's called the Freedom Care Unit, and it exists to help currently serving armed forces individuals who have either a chemical dependency problem and/or post-traumatic stress disorder related to their experiences in the military. There are only seventy beds, and the line of people who want to be admitted winds out the back door and clear around the building. Somebody leaves, and his bed doesn't have time to get cold. Soldiers bide their time in a number of various hospitals – either in the ER or on the few acute psych wards that are available – until they can get a bed placement with us.

Patients here are much more motivated. Oh, my goodness, are they polite and respectful. I get "Yes ma'am'd" to death. They want to work so hard, and the PTSD is really difficult for some of the young guys. I can remember one night, this young man couldn't sleep. It was the third time he'd been up and I said, "I could offer you meds, but maybe we can just sit and talk?" So I made him a cup of cocoa and we just sat down and he started verbally vomiting all of this ugly stuff. He had to get it out. As a nurse, it was so hard to sit there and listen to him describing the scene.

He had been a medic, and there was an explosion, and he was trying to pick his best friend up off the ground. As he put his hands underneath, his fingers literally entered the back of the man's skull. Underneath, where he couldn't see, the skull was shattered and his fingers slid right into his friend's brain matter. To this day, he can't eat anything that has that type of a texture. He was a paramedic; he couldn't help his best friend; he shouldn't have been the one who survived – it just went on and on and on. He couldn't stop talking about it.

I think I'm the first person he had trusted with his story. I don't want to take credit for anything other than this: that was the stage he had reached in his level of care, and I had the good sense to listen. He was finally able to get some of the horror out, and by no means had he resolved it all. He stayed there for another month and a half, working with the psychologist. Trauma doesn't evaporate just because you're in treatment. Sometimes you have to do disparate treatments, several different times, and continue for a long time on an out-patient basis.

But here's the thing: it's not only being able to listen, but to not register anything on your face. No approval, no disapproval. Just being there to take it in, because you don't know how anything you might say could affect someone in that state. Some people would say, "Oh, my God. That was a horrible thing." I just said to him, "You know, you didn't start out that day to deal with that issue. You put all of your knowledge into it, and you did everything you could to make it the best for your friend."

I believe he was in his twenties, and I'm in my fifties. I wasn't his mom, but I was someone who was close enough to representing that figure so he could feel safe telling me his terrible secret. In a situation like that, you really have to be careful and feel your way through it.

For me, being a mother to my children, and volunteering in Peru, and working as a nurse – they're all the same. They're my small ways of being responsible for the world, of giving back life. I would have adopted six dozen more kids, but I wouldn't have been effective as a parent with so many. You have to remember that there's only so much of you to go around. For the Peruvian kids, the chance to help them fix their hearts is the way I can give them a piece of my heart. That's what I can do there.

When I was a respiratory therapist, I only monitored part of the patient. As a nurse, I work with the whole patient, the entire person. The responsibility for each patient I have is sitting right on top of my shoulders. Not only do I have to watch for anything life-threatening, but I need to guide that person through the process of a disease. I also feel responsible for helping the family members and, along the way, it's especially important to offer education to everyone involved. I feel so fortunate that I have been given the opportunity to help people change their lives.

It doesn't always work, and I know that. Not everyone is going to listen. But if you've got the voice, and you can find the specific button that works with a particular patient, you can make all the difference in the world in that person's day. It's not an easy job and you have to care. You don't know if it's going to be the warm blanket that you put over them, the socks that you put on their toes when they're cold, or just being aware of their personal likes and dislikes. There is a place and a way for everybody to make a difference in another person's life. You just have to figure out what it is.

EKATERINA HUELSTER

I grew up in a small town in Russia. It's called Naberezhnye Chelny. I grew up with my mom. My father left us after he chose to have alcohol instead of a family. When I graduated from high school, I told my mom, "I want to be a nurse." And she said, "Okay." We have no relatives who were in the nursing profession. I entered medical college in 1998 in Russia, in my town.

I always wanted to help people. I always brought home sick cats and dogs and birds. In fact, I had a cat once that wasn't sick at all but I put bandages all over him, for no reason, just because I wanted to play at being a nurse. I always dressed up in white clothes, imagining they were my uniform. Maybe I felt like I was missing something in my life, like that love from my absent father. Instead of feeling sorry for myself, I focused my energy on becoming a nurse and helping people.

I entered the medical college and graduated in two years and ten months with ninety credits. I found a job in a critical care unit, and I was doing pretty well. I don't know if you're familiar with health care in Russia, but it's horrible. I'm not going to lie. In 1918, the Soviet Union was the first country to promise free universal health care. So we grew up with this idea: everybody deserves health care, at no cost. But that's not the reality. My mom is still in Russia and I am always thinking of how I can bring her here to America one day. Every time, when she goes to the doctor or she is admitted to the hospital, she needs to bring her own supplies. You basically can stay for free in the hospital, but supplies are your responsibility.

The hospital where I worked was awful. We basically had no hot water. And bribes, which you pay to the doctor, are normal. That is well known in Russia. There is no law that says doctors who take bribes will go to jail. In America, if you accept a bribe, forget it – the state can take your license away. In Russia, we recommend a doctor by saying, "Hey, you know what, I paid him and he took care of me."

My first client I will never ever forget. She had a heart problem, and I remember when I went to work that day, I asked, "Well, what kind of heart problem?" When they give a report in Russia, they're never specific. She was a female who had been complaining of chest pain, and she was about my mom's age back then, maybe fifty years old. Sure enough, within two days, the woman passed away. So I asked people why that happened. "Why did she die? Did she have a heart attack?" I was really upset, because when she died, no one even did an autopsy. The family just picked her up and made a funeral. If, in America, you die at such a young age from a heart problem that isn't specified, the family is going to ask what happened. They're going to demand some answers.

In Russia, when a patient goes to a hospital, he has nothing but hope. A patient just hopes he's going to make it, hopes he's not going to die, and hopes he's going to be okay.

After a year of working there, I didn't know what to do with my life. Every day I went to work in Russia, I was thinking, *Why am I a nurse? I do nothing good for people.*

Then, at the end of 2001, I told my mother, "I'm going to America." I actually believed that thing people say about the United States: it's a free country and the land of opportunity. But nobody tells you, before you go to America, that maybe you should learn to speak English. I didn't speak any English when I came here. Zero. It is a great country, if you have an education, if you have some relatives here, and if you have some money – not for somebody like me, who came here and had to live in the airport for a week.

I came after September 11, in 2002, on May 31. I was promised that someone would pick me up at the airport and drive me to the Kingsborough Community College in Brooklyn and that I could be a student there and learn English. Of course, that didn't happen. Nobody picked me up. I had $200 in my pocket. I didn't know the New York City area. I had no map. I don't know what I was thinking.

I stayed in the airport for one week. I slept at the gate. I washed my hair in the ladies room, ate any food I could find, drank water from the sink. There is a terminal for Aeroflot Company where people arrive from Moscow, and I found many Russian newspapers there. So I was reading those newspapers and looking for an apartment or room, and I started calling from a pay phone in the airport. The whole week I called people, and they were asking about my credit. But I had only been in

America a couple of days, and I hadn't left the airport. I didn't have any credit, and I knew nothing about all that.

Then I found a Russian family in the Brighton Beach area, and they had a room for rent for something like $100 a week, which I thought I could afford. And they said, "Yes, come here tomorrow," so I took a bus. However, my landlord drank a lot and I didn't feel safe there. The apartment was full of people who were doing strange activities, like selling drugs, and one guy worked for some company that was delivering girls to the nude clubs in New York City. There was constant drinking and arguing.

The only good thing was I understood Russian and I could protect myself, because I knew what they were talking about. They offered me drugs, but I never took them. They offered me a way to make easy money, which meant being a prostitute, and I was so shocked. I packed all my stuff in big garbage bags. You know those black garbage bags in America? I had never seen them before. I packed my stuff and I was out on the street again, looking for a new place to live. While walking around, I remember thinking to myself, It's not over yet. It's just a beginning. I can do this, and I will do this. I never looked back. I kept imagining that one day I would have a place to live, good food, an education, a job, a car, and a map of the United States.

I ended up living with another Russian family in the same area, Brighton Beach, and I took about twelve different jobs. I worked at pizza delivery. I worked by the ocean, where I had to separate the big fish from the small fish. It was all cash. So I got some jobs, but I got fired all the time. Like with pizza delivery, for example, I didn't know Brooklyn. I didn't have a car or a bicycle, and every time I tried to deliver a pizza, I would get lost. Of course, I never delivered the pizza, so I got fired. It was a terrible experience. I was just walking with the pizza, and I never understood those Brooklyn avenues which are designated in alphabetical order. I would always go in the wrong direction, or I would take the wrong train.

I also worked as a waitress in a restaurant – again, for cash. After I had saved my first $700.00, I took a bus, B1, and I went to Kingsborough Community College, because that was my original destination in the United States. I went there and I told them, "I need to learn English. I have $700 cash. Can I pay, and could you please teach me English?" So they put me into the English as a Second Language program. I was taking the B1 bus every morning, and it took about fifty minutes to get there. Then I got tired of living in that place, because I had nothing but sad experiences in Brooklyn. I thought, *Why don't I move to New Jersey?*

So I moved, rented a room, and kept working. I entered Union County College in New Jersey and continued to learn English. When I understood English a little better, I spoke with the people at the college, and I said, "I was a nurse in Russia. How can I be a nurse in America?" They just stared at me. "You have to take the NCLEX, but you're not going to be able to understand the scientific language."

And I said, "Okay, so I can't be a nurse?"

"No, you have to go back to nursing school and start over."

I told myself, *You have two choices: you can give up on your life and go back to Russia and maybe even accept the bribes. Or you're going to stay here and make something better of your life, and maybe you can bring your mom here someday.* I decided to start from the very beginning because I wanted to be a nurse so badly.

I graduated on August 23, 2005, from Union County College, and I have a diploma on my wall at home stating that I can speak English. If you're not born in this country, you have to go to this kind of program before you get accepted into college. Learning English was for me a green light to continue pursuing my dreams. I continued to study and took every prerequisite class before being accepted into a traditional nursing school, and I stayed there for two years, but that was a very challenging time for me.

I had heard about a "distance" nursing program for adults with health care experience like me, and I decided to apply there. I was not only accepted, but they also allowed me to skip some exams because I had good grades in previous nursing classes. I graduated in less than a year. I passed all my exams. I never failed one. Then I had to pass a three-day clinical competency assessment, where I demonstrated all my knowledge. In seven months, I was done. When I received my nursing diploma, I was crying so hard. I couldn't believe all my hard work had paid off.

After I had completed my bachelor's component of the RN-MS program, in 2008, the economy hurt health care facilities and many nurses were laid off. There was a lot of competition for experienced nurses in New Jersey, and new grads were left out of the picture. So I started to work in adult medical care. It wasn't my dream job. The patients I worked with were the elderly who couldn't stay home alone. Most of it was basic stuff, not really like hospital experience. It was medical care where you come to work at eight in the morning and you leave at four in the afternoon, because that's when the family members picked the clients up or a bus delivered them back home.

Currently, I am a hospice nurse, and I love it. I work with patients who prefer to stay with their families in their own homes until the last moment, but some of them live in nursing homes or assisted-living places. I can't explain why, but a connection exists between me and hospice patients. Maybe it's because I know how someone feels when they are about to lose a loved one. I feel their pain, emptiness, anger, and numbness. I stand by them and listen to them. I am present there for them. I never thought that I could find such rewarding feelings through hospice. I have learned valuable information from my own life events, and that makes me not only a compassionate nurse, but also a friend for my patients and their families. Right now I'm still in school and looking forward to getting my master's degree so I can become a hospice nurse educator.

Let's say something magical happens in the health care system in Russia. I still would never ever want to go back there as a nurse. Something was broken for me back when I first wanted to do good for people. I think every nurse in America should be thankful that they have such a wonderful opportunity. They should go to work, not like, "Oh, I have to go do my job now," but they should think, *I'm going to go and make a difference in somebody else's life and that makes me so happy every day.* America permits me to live my life to the fullest, to dream without limits, to deliver kindness and service to my patients, and to simply enjoy being a nurse here.

DR. SHELLEY MORISTON

I have been a nurse since 1985, serving first in the U. S. Army and then as a civilian. I am currently completing my second doctoral degree in Nursing Education, and I am under contract with McGraw-Hill Publishers to write a book on psychiatric nursing. In February 2012, I was appointed Dean of the Denver School of Nursing.

I went into the Army right out of high school. I was on delayed entry for a year. I actually joined in 1983, the summer before my senior year. I saw where my friends were going and I didn't want to go there. I'm from Iowa, and I knew I didn't want to stay there and work at a Hardee's or at the mall. I wanted to have a life and a career. I actually joined to be a linguist originally, and then they didn't have enough people signed up to teach the class, so they offered me an alternative as a medic. That started it for me. I just fell in love with health care.

Initially, I became a nurse because I was so impressed with all the male nurses I saw there. That's what inspired me – all those military officers. They were so professional and smart. This was at a time when it was still unusual for men to pick nursing as a profession. I had never seen male nurses before, and I thought, I want to be one of them. There were so many incredible role models that it just opened doors for me I never even knew about.

These guys were determined to continue their educations. They weren't content to have earned just bachelor's degrees. They were all going to school for their master's, and they all wanted to really shine so they could work in the high-intensity areas of the hospital –the ER and the ICU and the trauma unit. Ultimately, I did the same thing. When I worked as a medic, I absolutely did feel like, *Here is where I'm supposed to be, and this is what I'm supposed to be doing.* I understood that as far back as when I was a medic and I was applying to LPN school.

My father passed away a couple of years ago, but he was always so very proud of me for being a medic in the Army and then becoming a nurse. He was a preacher, and he always talked about the calling. "Sometimes the calling isn't as obvious as you want it to be," he would say. "Sometimes it takes a little while for it to happen." He told me that some people know from birth what they're going to be, and they know they've gotten the calling, or the message. It didn't work that way for me.

My dad is actually the reason I ultimately heard my "calling" to become a nurse. It came much later in my life, but it sure came strong, and I know there's nothing else in the world that I'd want to be. I thought then, This is the right thing. This is my journey. And I did feel called at that point.

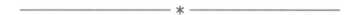

After I finished my year of LPN training in Tacoma, Washington, I was sent to Ireland Army Hospital at Fort Knox, Kentucky. I got transferred to a blood dyscrasia ward, and this was at the time when AIDS was really peaking. People were dying literally within days of being diagnosed. The disease didn't even have a name then. I got assigned to that ward, and when I first arrived, I got freaked out and didn't want to do it.

This was 1986 in Kentucky, and they just didn't know much about AIDS. We had some soldiers who didn't acknowledge at that time they were gay, but with some of them you could tell. But that wasn't the only population in which the disease manifested. We had one woman who had gotten it from her husband, we treated children born with it there, and we saw several elderly hemophiliacs who had become infected by blood transfusions. These all occurred in that time before they knew the virus was in the blood. Nobody knew anything about it, and I was certainly afraid of getting it.

However, I watched hospital staff members ignoring patients because of their similar fears, and it just made me go totally the opposite way. I know this will sound a little corny, but I thought of Florence Nightingale when she was in the Crimean War. Almost all of the nurses that she originally took with her died, because they said they didn't care that the patients had communicable diseases. They were there to care for them. I thought, *You know, if I get sick, then I get sick. But I'm here to care for these people.* So I did it, and it was actually life-changing for me. It helped me realize that I'm not doing this for me. I'm doing it for other people, and I can't be afraid of this disease.

Then we had these infant twins who were born with AIDS. This was just after I was discharged from the Army, when I had begun working as a pediatric home health nurse, and I was involved in a new pilot program at the local hospital. Nurses who cared for children in the hospital were also assigned to those same children after they were sent home. We were also responsible for teaching foster parents how to care for their new children. Well, the family that was going to foster those twins with AIDS backed out, and I got that case. I actually volunteered for it, and I just fell in love with those little babies. They were so cute. Nobody wanted them. They only weighed two pounds each. I'd sit and hold them in my lap and they'd play with my nose. It just really made me stop being afraid, and I needed that.

In the end, of course, it became terribly sad. They both passed while I was caring for them, and I was with each of them when they died. It was really hard for me – in fact, probably one of my hardest experiences ever. But I also loved it. I tell my students about it now. I tell that story because it's such a powerful part of being a nurse: you get to be the very first person that someone sees when he emerges from the womb, and sometimes you get to be the very last to hold his hand as he leaves this world. We knew that those twins weren't going to live very long, but my role as a nurse was to love them until they passed, and to be with them all the way until the very end. And I was. That was one of the best gifts I ever received.

Nurses are unlike any other health care workers in the hospital. You can really connect with patients, at quite a profound level. You have an opportunity to share yourself with them, but they also share themselves with you because it's such an intimate experience for them. I found that to be incredible. I thought at one point that maybe I should go on and train to be a physician, so I started watching the doctors. I realized pretty quickly, though, that they weren't offered the same opportunities that I was given on a daily basis. They didn't get to establish the bond with the patient that a nurse enjoys, and they didn't get to be a part of the challenges that patients have to face. So I decided I wanted to stay a nurse.

*

In 1989, I got a scholarship – it was called a Green to Gold Scholarship – while I was still stationed at Fort Knox. It was an active-duty scholarship to attend Vanderbilt University. When I originally got the scholarship,

Vanderbilt offered a baccalaureate degree in nursing. Then, when I actually went there to begin school in 1989, they had changed their program and no longer offered that bachelor's program. They had created what's called a bridge program, so that you started with whatever credits you had and worked continuously until you completed the master's degree. I was in that program from 1989 until 1991, and I was in ROTC that whole time as well. But I didn't complete the master's degree because I ran out of money.

The scholarship from the Army paid only a small percentage of my college costs, and Vanderbilt was very expensive – $575 a credit hour when I started, and it went up every year. When I left in 1991, it was $775 a credit hour. Everything cost so much in Nashville. I was living out of my car. I had an apartment, but I never had time to go home. I literally was going from job to job to school to job. I had one of those little wind-up clocks and I would sleep in my car and set it. My load was eighteen to twenty hours every term. I was out of my league, drowning. I struggled for two years there, and that was it.

By 1991, I knew I needed to pull out of the program and regroup. That's why I looked at Regents College. I thought, *Why don't I just do the associate's degree, and then I can always get the bachelor's after I finish that? And eventually I can go on for the master's, instead of trying to go for the whole thing all at once.* I did have all my credits, and they transferred, and I had also taken a few classes over at Tennessee State University, and they were accepted by Regents as well. I started in the beginning of 1994 and I graduated in '96 with my associate's degree.

During that time, I was working critical care for three different nursing agencies in Nashville, so I was floating all over the city. Then I got a job working at a clinic, and as soon as I graduated from Regents, they made me director of nursing for that clinic. That became my first job as an RN. But almost immediately I decided I wanted to do something very different.

I had heard about this place in Antioch, Tennessee, that served children with profound developmental disabilities. It was a cluster facility where they had little cottages that were in the shape of a "U" on the property. I went there and interviewed and, as it would happen, a friend was the assistant director of nursing there. So I took the job. It was a place called Mur-Ci Homes, and they admitted children ages three to sixteen who were medically fragile. Some of them were so fragile they could barely even be turned. Sometimes families just seemed to dump them and never came back. I had never worked with that population, and I instantly fell in love with those kids. I became so enraptured with developmental-disabilities nursing that I joined the Developmental Disabilities Nursing Association, and I became certified. That was the first certification I got as an RN.

After that, I began to steer my career toward other vulnerable populations. I really have spent my whole career working with the neediest patients. I transitioned from developmental disability into traumatic and acquired brain injuries. I stayed with that population for a while, and then I started working with psychiatric mental health patients, especially with pervasive mental illness – the really, truly ill. I became involved with forensics and with the criminally insane who were definitive sociopathic personalities. Caring for those that others don't want to care for has really been my life's work. Those are the people I seek out. When I'm looking for a job, I look for places where others don't want to be, and that's exactly where I find a home. I don't know why. Maybe I'm just drawn to the underdog.

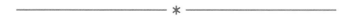

Right before coming here to the college, I served as the Director of Nursing in the state psychiatric hospital at Fort Logan in Denver, Colorado. The patients there are mostly indigent, and it's a very old facility. Many of the patients have pervasive mental illness, and some of them have lived there for twenty years. They're just intractable. You really aren't going to resolve their conditions. They're never going to be able to live a normal life in the community. Most nurses just don't want to work with those seemingly hopeless patients and, once again, I was drawn to it.

As director of nursing, I would sometimes go to individual patient meetings, where I could listen to the staff and could do some mentoring. I would help them brainstorm different care options for people. When the team felt stuck – when they as if like they had tried everything with a patient and they just didn't know where to go – that was when I would say, "Well, have you thought about this?" I could function as a new set of eyes for them.

For example, we had a fourteen-year-old who had complex catatonia. He was completely unresponsive. He had been catatonic for about eight months, and it wasn't his first time. This was his longest period, though, and his parents were really worried. He needed total care. He was no longer eating. He had to be fed through a nasal gastric tube, and the team felt like there was nothing more that they could do. They were ready to give up. They had tried every conceivable drug to try and bring this kid out of it, and nothing had worked.

I had just completed electro-convulsive therapy training to be an ECT nurse, and we had an ECT suite there. So I brought it up. I said, "Have we thought about this? We've used it before for adults with catatonia who were intractable, and it was very successful."

That became a big ethical issue, because they had never done it with an adolescent before. I said, "Don't you think that he deserves, at least, that we try this? If nothing else is working, rather than give up, is there any reason why we shouldn't try? Is there any risk to him that is so severe that we can't give him this chance?"

So I did a lot of research on it, and I found several cases where it had been done in other places, at other times in history, and it had been successful. I brought those to the team, and I really worked with them to get past their reservations. We spoke with the parents and explained the risks versus the benefits. They were so despondent at that point, after eight months of their child being totally absent, that they agreed.

I was one of the ECT nurses during the procedure. Immediately after the boy received his very first treatment, within seconds of the procedure, he sat up on the gurney and looked at each person, eye to eye, and he said, "I'm hungry." Those were his first words in eight months. Well, everybody started laughing, and he didn't understand what was so funny. He didn't realize that he had been essentially unconscious for all that time.

Well, let me tell you, he ended up becoming a holy terror. He tore the whole place up. His behavior was out of control. It was a rough patch for a while there, after he came out of it. In the end, when he left the hospital, he was back on track, balanced, on medication, going back to school, and doing really well. We had achieved a success, again, by overcoming our fears and trying something we hadn't tried before. That hospital has incredibly devoted nurses and physicians. They provide outstanding care in spite of the outdated facilities, and I enjoyed my work there very much.

——————————— ✳ ———————————

The one patient that I'll never forget was a young man who had AIDS. It was at a skilled nursing home where I went, under contract, through a nursing agency in Nashville.

He was only twenty-four, and I don't remember his name, but you could tell that he had been a really good-looking young man before he got the disease. But he was just absolutely eaten up with Kaposi's Sarcoma. The lesions were actually right on top of each other and scaling. He really did look a little monstrous, and the staff that worked at the facility didn't want to care for him. They would take his bedside table, pull it over to the door, place his food tray on it, and then push it toward his bed. They wouldn't even go in and feed him, and he was so weak that he couldn't feed himself. I thought that was just so cruel.

I was under contract as the charge nurse, and the first time I saw that, I told the CNAs, "That is not acceptable, and you're not going to do it while I'm here." I did the whole lecture spiel. But I also wanted them to see me model good behavior, so I went in and sat on the edge of the bed, pulled the tray over, took the top off, and started feeding the guy. I was talking away to him about how beautiful the day was and how, after he finished eating, I would take him for a shower if he wanted one. Then we could go outside for a walk, which meant me pushing him around the grounds of the facility in his wheelchair. He was just too weak to walk at that point.

He had already been there for a month. There he was, dying – he probably only had three weeks left. He was in hospice. His whole family had disowned him, so he had nobody. And then the CNAs were treating him like that because they were scared of him. It just broke my heart. All of a sudden, I realized he was crying, because I was the first person who had spoken to him since he had been there. He couldn't believe I had sat down on his bed and that I was talking to him and feeding him. So we ended up becoming great friends for those last three weeks of his life. Every day, I was the one who gave him his shower. Every day, I was the one who fed him his breakfast. Every day, I took him outside for a walk.

I'd even make sure I sped up my med-pass in the morning so I would have more time with him. I tried to make the final days fun for him.

I discovered that he loved books, and I've been an antiquarian book collector my whole life. His vision had deteriorated so much as a part of the disease process that he was no longer able to read, and books on tape were not common then the way they are today. So I brought in a book every day and, at the end of my shift, I would read to him. Then he and I would discuss what I had read. I could tell that he looked forward to our times together. He really started to open up to me. He told me about his life and how hard things had been for him since becoming ill with AIDS. His life partner at the time had dumped him and left him with no place to live; he had been fired from his job; and his family had abandoned him. He literally had nothing and no one. He was truly and utterly alone, and dying that way.

I had the privilege of being with him when he left this world. I was sitting on his bed, holding his hand. He looked me in the eyes and a small tear rolled down his left cheek. Then he gently squeezed my hand. The last words he said were spoken to me: "Thank you." He died, of course, but at least he died almost at peace. I know that sounds funny, but he wasn't afraid anymore, and he wasn't alone. I have to admit that I went home and cried for three days as I mourned that loss. But if I had it to do again, I would do everything exactly the same way.

Nurses do so much with their minds, and they are so engaged in technology today, that they sometimes forget the most healing tool we possess in our arsenal is simple human touch. I really try to instill in my students the importance of being in the moment with your patients and using human touch to be one with them. Studies have shown time and again that human touch speeds healing and reduces anxiety in patients. I have certainly seen the power of it in my career as a nurse.

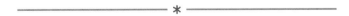

I've had so many incredible experiences. Besides being with that young man who died of AIDS or with those two little babies, I think maybe the best thing that has happened to me is what I'm going through right now, here, with this college. Denver School of Nursing has only been open since

2004. We're a young college, so we're just finalizing our accreditation, and I've been doing a lot of work around that. As the new dean, I have to make sure that the schedules are being followed and all assignments are completed. I conduct classroom observations of faculty, and I do a lot of student advising, as well. I handle all the transcript reviews for transfer credit for the college. I write all the letters welcoming people who have been accepted and, of course, there are lots and lots of meetings.

I'm pretty ambitious, and I have trouble with one little word: "No." For some reason, I can't say it. I think that's part of being a nurse. We don't usually say no. I observe my faculty, and they share the same problem. Because I can't say no, during my time here, I've taught almost every course that the college offers. I don't mean to toot my horn, but I feel as if I've been able to accomplish so much and to really move this school to a level that's unbelievable. I tell you, I can't imagine doing anything else in my life right now. After almost thirty years as a nurse, this is where I want to be, where I'm supposed to be. There was this great quote by Mother Teresa. She said, "Believe that you are exactly where you are meant to be." And I think that expresses how I feel right now.

I tell my students that the wonderful thing about nursing is, if you don't like some area or you get a little burned out in it, you can go to another. You can try new things. You don't have to be afraid. It's a great profession. It's so much more than a profession, and I talk to my students about that, too. It's an art. It truly is an art. I have a kind of credo that I created and I have it posted on my office door at the college. I also say it when I speak at commencement ceremonies, because I truly believe it:

> *Above all else, know that nursing is not solely a science, but so, too, an art worthy of mastery, inspiration, and admiration. We are all truly students of the art for life, and we each continually strive to be better today than we were yesterday. Be mindful of the talents of others around you. Rather than envy their abilities, emulate them and grow through your knowing of them. This is the TRUE spirit of a nurse.*

REBECCA SWEET

I came to nursing late in my life. Even though I've known since I was six years old that I wanted to be a nurse, I didn't become an RN until I turned sixty. I was an LPN for a couple of years before that. Now I work as a case manager for a hospice company in Albuquerque, New Mexico, and I couldn't be happier.

Sometimes I hesitate to tell people this story because I'm afraid they'll think I'm crazy. It wasn't like I was hearing voices. It was more like a telegram from God to my heart, and that message told me I needed to go back to nursing school. I didn't want to hear that. Now I wouldn't say I'm a particularly religious person, but I am very spiritual. I have a connection with nature, and a connection with God through nature and through my relationships with other people. But I felt alone at that point. My life was falling apart and I frankly didn't know from day to day whether I wanted to be alive, let alone undertake something like nursing school again. I was so tired and depressed, and I said, "No, God, I'm sorry. I can't do that." Well, God wouldn't be quiet. She just kept saying, *You know this is what you need to do. You've always known that you wanted to be a nurse, and this is the time. If you don't do it now, when are you going to do it?*

The nurse part rang true. I think I knew by the time I was six years old that nursing was what I wanted to do. I was always asking for those little nursing kits with the little bag, and my mother would say, "They don't make nursing bags. They make doctor bags." I would tell her, "I don't want a doctor bag. I want a nursing bag, with a lot of bandages and some adhesive tape." And of course the stethoscope. I didn't mention that, but I believed any legitimate nursing bag had to contain one of those.

I went to nursing school the first time when I was twenty-six. I was married at that time, living in Oklahoma City, and we had a daughter who was four. I was enrolled full time in a two-year diploma program that was offered by a Catholic hospital in Oklahoma City. I made it through the first year, doing very well academically, but I was burning out. Trying to be a full-time wife and mother and student, all at the same time, was too much, and I didn't have a strong support system. I went in to tell my instructors I was going to quit the program and they tried to talk me out of it. They said, "Why don't you take some time off and rest and then come back. Just please don't quit." And I said, "Well, what's going to be different when I come back? Nothing is going to change."

So I quit and I went off in another direction. By then I was divorced and my daughter lived with her father. I remarried, and my second husband was a philosophy professor at a university in Kansas. Most of his family worked in education: his father was a professor; his mother and brother were teachers; his brother's wife was a teacher. I thought, *Well, in order to fit into this family, I better be an academic.*

I enrolled in a university and got both my bachelor's and my master's degrees in English, and then earned a second bachelor's in geography just for fun. And after that I was accepted into the University of Oklahoma's Ph.D. in English program with a focus on Native American Studies, but they changed the requirements once I had moved there and started my courses. They said I was going to have to stay an extra year and do student teaching. I asked why, and they said I needed the experience. I said, "I've already been teaching at the university in Kansas. I don't really need that." And they said, "Sorry, we've changed the program, and that's a part of our requirements now." So back to Kansas I went, and stayed there for twenty-four years, teaching but also serving as an administrative assistant to one of the deans.

By the end of 2006, it was clear my life was out of control. I thought, *Okay, my marriage is falling apart. I hate where I live. I hate my job. I feel like I'm living my life for nothing.* And to be honest, I was drinking pretty heavily and was very depressed. It was hell. There's no other way to put it.

For Christmas that year, my husband went to visit his family in Colorado. I told him I couldn't go, and he went without me. It was within that two-week period – when he was gone and I was alone – that I got the calling. I was of course still drinking, so every night I was getting drunk and sitting in front of the fireplace, sobbing and crying my heart out, and having these strange conversations with God. Finally, I just gave up and said out loud, "Okay. All right. If you're calling me to do this, I'll do it. But you're going to have to help me, because I can't do this alone."

When my husband got back, I told him that I was going to quit my job and go to nursing school, because God was calling me to do that. And he said, "I can't see that ever happening." Remember, he was a philosophy professor, so his head was constantly in the clouds. If it hadn't been, he probably would have tried to get me committed somewhere.

I was still working at the university, but the first thing I needed to do was get my CNA certificate so I could have that experience before I went into nursing school. I didn't really have a plan. I just knew that this was what God wanted me to do, and I had to do it, so I started night classes to become a CNA.

In September 2007, I left my husband. I packed my car and moved out. I continued to work at the university until January 2008, when I took early retirement. I had been working there for so long that I didn't have to resign. Then I took a position as an aide for hospice. It was a tremendous pay cut from my university job. Physically, it was messy, stressful, hard work, and there was a lot of driving because our hospice covered a fifty-mile area, but I was so happy. I completely loved it. And I knew that I was on the right track, so I continued. I applied for the LPN program at Johnson County Community College in Kansas City and was accepted. I finished there in May 2009.

I had always been fascinated with the Southwest and with Native American cultures, so I got on a train and rode out to Albuquerque during my next Christmas break. Immediately I fell in love with the place. I didn't know a soul there, and I didn't have a job at that point. But I got in touch with a real estate agent, and I told her, "I want you to help me find a place, because I want to move out here." We looked and looked and finally she took me to a village called Corrales, which is a suburb of Albuquerque and was actually founded by hippies back in the 1970s, and I said, "This is it. I don't have to look any further." I put down a deposit on a condo and went back to Kansas to finish my nursing program, knowing I was going to move to Albuquerque when I got out.

When I went through my LPN program, there were thirty-three of us in my class. There was a moment at the beginning of the school year when they asked us to get up and tell the other students a little bit about our background and what kind of nursing we wanted to do. I was the only one who said she wanted to do hospice nursing. Everyone reacted: "Oh, that's gross," or "That's so depressing," or "Why do you want to do that?"

I told them that when I got my call to go into nursing, I knew that hospice was what I needed to do. I was sure I could handle the physical aspects of dying. It may sound weird but, now, sometimes I'm not really even depressed by it. It makes me sad when I see a young person die, of course, but hospice is really so different from what we were taught in nursing school, where you're taught to help people heal and send them home to continue their lives. With hospice, that's not the point. The reality is that your patient won't get better. This person is dying and has chosen to seek palliative care rather than aggressive treatment. Our job is to go into the home or the facility and to make sure they're comfortable, to help them die with dignity, and to comfort their families.

However, I couldn't get a job in hospice when I first moved to Albuquerque. Out here, most of the hospices don't hire LPNs, so I tried my best to find a position in a retirement community or a nursing home. Nobody was hiring. Finally, I accepted a position at the municipal detention center, and I worked the midnight shift at the jail as an infirmary nurse. That was interesting.

I didn't have any trouble at all working with the inmates. They were, for the most part, respectful of the nurses, as long as they thought the nurses were actually there to help them. Some of the nurses were tough to work with, though, because they thought of the inmates as the scum of the earth and treated them that way. I had more trouble working with some of my colleagues than I did with the inmates. But what it finally came down to was that I had trouble working nights. At my age, I couldn't get my body to switch from a day rhythm to a night rhythm, and I started getting sick. I lasted two months and learned a lot, but then I got a call from a retirement community.

I switched over and worked there for fifteen months. I really loved that job, and I got close to many of the residents. I adore old people. They are so out there, the way a lot of children are. They'll say whatever they're thinking, and if they feel like crap, they'll say that. And if they think you look like crap, they'll tell you that, too. I just love their honesty. Finally, I had to quit because I was in a car accident and broke my foot. I couldn't walk my rounds anymore. However, while I was working there at the retirement community, one of my residents said to me, "You could have been a doctor." And I answered, "Well, maybe I could have been a doctor, but I never wanted to set my sights that low."

I didn't mean to disparage doctors with that comment. What I meant was I don't think most doctors can develop the kinds of relationships with their patients that nurses can. Doctors have to get in and out so quickly these days. They're so overworked that they really can't spend the time getting to know their patients. The most important thing in my life is establishing intimate connections with people, and nursing allows me to do that. But I realized right then that I had to become an RN to have what I truly wanted as a nurse.

I took a temporary desk job, working for another hospice company here in Albuquerque as a continuous quality-improvement coordinator, while my foot healed and while I completed my course work for my RN. On February 21, 2012, the day before my 60th birthday, I took the NCLEX for my RN and passed it, which was surprising to me because it was so difficult. I logged onto the state board of nursing website later the same day and they already had my license up there. I was so happy, I cried. I couldn't believe that I had passed. It was posted there, my RN license, and it said, REBECCA SWEET, Registered Nurse, and I literally jumped up and down, which isn't so easy to do when you have a broken foot. That was probably the happiest day of my life.

Soon after that, I was fortunate enough to get my job as a case manager at Ambercare Hospice. This is a great company with warm, loving people, whose hearts are in this business. It's an employee-owned company, so we're also working for our own good as we're helping clients. The case managers are in charge of coordinating the care for all their patients, and they are the point persons for the entire team. We collaborate with the physician, pharmacy, medical equipment providers, social worker, chaplain, aide, and the volunteer and bereavement coordinators. It's hard, but I love the responsibility, and I love knowing that these people trust me and respect me.

I work Monday through Friday, 8:00 a.m. to 5:00 p.m., making patient visits. We're required to see the patients at least once a week, but if they're very ill or actively dying, then we go more often. I'll go every day for a visit if they're active, to make sure that their symptoms are being controlled. I do all of my charting on the computer. All of us have laptops that we take with us everywhere and do our documentation for the patient on site. I occasionally have to go into the office to pick up supplies, consult with another team member, or talk over a patient's care with my manager. Most of the time, I'm making patient visits, speaking to the physician, ordering durable medical equipment, or setting up med profiles and ordering medications. If a patient lives way out in the boonies, where the pharmacy doesn't deliver, I'll go pick the meds up and deliver them myself.

When you're with people as they're dying, you develop an honest connection with them that I think is pretty rare in our society. To develop any kind of intimate connection with anyone is hard because we're all in such a hurry to do things, to go places, and to get things done. Our society focuses more on wealth, on talent, and on ownership of material possessions than on relationships. But hospice offers opportunities for deeper meaning.

I often feel a presence in the room when I'm with somebody who is dying. I had a patient who passed over the weekend and, because I was one of the on-call nurses, I went to make the pronouncement. Even though he was one of my patients, he was unresponsive the whole time I had known him. However, I had gotten to know his wife, his three daughters, and his son pretty well. They were all there at his bedside for the last three days of his life.

The first thing that happened when I walked in the door was that they were all there, thanking me for coming. They all lined up and hugged me. I went in and pronounced him, and I asked them if they wanted me to call the funeral home or if they wanted to do that. They asked me to do it, but then they said they weren't ready for them to come yet. "Is it okay if we stay with him for a while?" And I said, "Of course."

One of his daughters was a beautician, a stylist, and she said, "Could I get my clippers and trim his beard? He would have hated the way he looks. I don't want him to go off to the funeral home looking like that." And I said, "Absolutely."

She trimmed his beard, and then I asked them, "Would you like me to prepare the body – to wash him and to change his clothes?" And they said they'd like that very much. So I asked them to leave the room, because I have to do some things that I don't like the family to witness, and I began to wash his body. While I was doing that, his son, who was probably in his forties, came into the room and said, "Is there anything that I can help you with?" And I said, "You know, you're welcome to be here and do anything you want. Please don't stay if you're uncomfortable." And he said, "No, I want to be here."

At one point, I asked him to help me turn his father's body to the side so I could wash his back. There are things that go on with bodies, like rigor mortis, or dependent lividity, and his father had been dead long enough that lividity was beginning. When we rolled him to the side, he saw that, and I said, "If this is bothering you, go ahead and step out. I can do it." But he repeated, "No, I want to be here."

He helped me finish bathing him. Then he sat in a chair by the bed and started sobbing. I felt God in the room at that time, because he was able to achieve some closure. I stood there quietly and let him sob. A lot of times I don't offer to comfort people when they're crying because I've had people pat me on the back and say, "There there, don't cry," and things like that. That's not what I want to hear when I'm crying. I covered his father up with a blanket, crossed his hands over his chest, and let his son cry.

It's humbling that people allow me to come into their homes and do this for their loved ones. They'll allow me to stand there and be with them while they're expressing their deepest emotions. To how many people in your life do you show those raw emotions?

I think maybe my need to feel this intimate connection with people was born out of my relationship with my maternal grandmother. She was my closest friend when I was little. I grew up in a home where my father's storms of rage crashed over our heads all the time. For some of my childhood, we lived next door to my grandmother, who lived in an actual log cabin in Tahlequah, Oklahoma. Whenever my father exploded, I would flee to my grandmother's. She'd sit me down at her kitchen table, which had one of those red-and-white-checked, oilcloth tablecloths, and give me milk and graham crackers, or candy orange slices and say, "Well, let's go out in the garden for a while." And we'd go out and hoe weeds. She always had hollyhocks and old-fashioned flowers like peonies, as well as vegetables. I always loved being outside with her. I loved being anywhere with her. She was such a calming presence – kind and gentle and loving. She always accepted me for who I was and never asked me to be anything else.

I feel like I'm serving God through the work that I do. And yet, is it hard? Yes, it's hard. It's always difficult to be around someone who's dying and whose family is grieving.

I was taking care of this one woman who said, "I know that I'm dying. I'm ready. I don't want to do this anymore." She was completely calm, drained from the chemo she had recently stopped. So I lay down on the bed next to her and kissed her bald head. "My job is to be here for you and to do everything I can do to keep you comfortable," I told her. "You've told me you just want to be comfortable until you die, and so that's what we're doing. I'll do everything I can not to let you down."

A lot of nurses don't like dealing with the interpersonal aspects of nursing. I've heard many nurses say things like, "It's exciting to be an ER nurse," or "You learn the most as an operating room nurse," or "I want to work in a doctor's office where I'm doing nothing but procedures." Well, in those kinds of jobs, you don't really connect with people a lot, because you don't spend that much time with them. You don't get the opportunity to build deep and meaningful relationships with those patients. Building those relationships is what nursing is all about. After all, what am I going to take with me when I die? Nothing material. More importantly, what am I going to leave behind that will be of value? I believe the only thing I can leave behind is someone's memory of me and what it meant for them to know me, and that's enough.

KATHY BROWNE

I have been an oncology nurse for thirty-one years. Until August 2012, I was the clinical coordinator of the oncology unit at North Florida Regional Medical Center in Gainesville. However, I felt I was getting further and further away from patient care, so I stepped down to work again as a staff nurse in oncology on the night shift.

For some mysterious reason, cancer has been an integral part of my life. My great aunt had cancer and I can remember as a child going to visit her. She just had this wide, black spot where her forehead should have been. It was necrotic, I'm sure. I was very young, but I remember being fascinated by it. Strange the things you remember. I meet with all the new students who work on our unit, and the first thing I tell them is, "The best thing that ever happened to me was cancer because, if I had never gotten cancer, I wouldn't be a nurse." And that's the truth.

I'm from Staten Island, and my first job after high school was with the General Services Administration, the one they have on the news all the time. At that time, I was having some health problems. I had this funny growth in my throat, and it was pushing out of my neck. I kept going to the doctor, but he didn't take it seriously. "Look, you're twenty years old," he told me. "You're a hypochondriac. There's nothing wrong with you."

What I really wanted back then was to be a CPA, and when I landed a job in a financial planning office on Wall Street, I thought, This is a great way to get my foot in the door. I had to get a physical for that job, and it just happened that the man who did my physical was an endocrinologist. He took one look at my neck and said, "Do you realize that you have a severe thyroid condition?" One look, before he had even examined me, and he knew. He looked at my eyes, felt my neck, and he said, "It's your thyroid. I can tell."

What I had was papillary carcinoma with a follicular component – a really strange type of thyroid cancer – but nobody told me that for a while, even though my parents knew. I was crying all the time. I had lost thirty pounds, and I just wasn't functioning properly. So he recommended another endocrinologist, who decided that I definitely needed surgery.

When I got to the hospital, I was supposed to have a private room. I went into the waiting room, and a nun was sitting there. She had thyroid cancer, too, and there was this giant goiter on her neck. Mine was small, but hers was huge. They were arguing with her in the admitting department, telling her that she had to go into a semi-private room. Being Catholic, I knew that nuns needed privacy and, because I had a private room, I told them, "Look, give her my room. I'll go in a semi-private room. I really don't care."

Later that night, I decided I would go visit her. I was fascinated by her condition. I thought it was really weird that this woman had a giant growth on her neck. I went to talk to her and passed out in her doorway. The nurses deposited me in a wheelchair and wheeled me back to my room. They said if I got out of bed one more time, they would restrain me.

This was in 1977, and there was no oncology unit in that hospital. I was on a regular surgical floor. My nurses were probably only a year or so older than I was, and they provided no teaching prior to my surgery. So when I woke up in my room after the operation, I had a wide stabilizing band around my neck, and I had no idea what it was. I crawled down to the end of the bed to read a suspicious-looking bottle. Years ago, the betadyne and the trach set were kept in glass bottles in case of emergencies, but no one had explained that, either. So I picked up the bottle and yelled, "You're not sticking this thing in my neck," and I hurled it against the wall. Well, the nurses weren't too happy with me from the night before when I passed out, and after I smashed some of their equipment, they treated me even worse.

After my recuperation, I went back to my job on Wall Street. On my first day there, the vice president called me into his office. He closed the door and said, "You have cancer. You're going to die. Why don't you just quit?" I was more than angry. I thought, *I just found out that nurses are awful people, and now I'm being told that I should quit because I might die someday.*

I left work, went home, and announced to my parents, "I'm going to nursing school." Everybody looked at me like I was crazy, and my mom said, "You couldn't even pass science in high school. You're just not good at that kind of stuff." And I answered, "I'm going to become a nurse and take care of cancer patients so people don't get treated the same way I was." I had been pretty wild as a teenager, so naturally my parents didn't think I'd stick with it. But I graduated from nursing school, got my RN license in 1981, and thirty-one years later, here I am, still an oncology nurse.

A funny thing happened when I went in for an interview for my first nursing job. The Director of Nurses met with every new nurse, and she said to me, "Now tell me, what would you like to do here?"

"I'd like to work in oncology," I told her.

"My God," she said, "I've been a nurse for thirty years, and you're the first nurse who has ever requested oncology."

I looked at her and thought, *What's so strange about that?* Then she admitted, "It's where I usually stick someone who doesn't get what she wants."

She did give me what I asked for, oncology, and I learned a lot. One of my earliest patients was a woman who had the most awful colon cancer. She had fistulas everywhere, openings all over her, and they drained stool throughout her whole body. We'd have to put her in the shower, and I'd climb in there with her and scrub her clean. There was no other way to do it. She had worked for a big hotel chain that had its own cookbook and, before she died, she gave me a copy of that cookbook, and she autographed it for me. I still use it today, and I think about her whenever I do.

But I had always hated the cold in New York, so I knew I wouldn't last there. I decided I wanted to live in the South. And during my first year in that oncology job, my husband and I had gotten divorced, so that cut one more tie. Then my best friend's parents moved to Dunedin, Florida, just north of Clearwater Beach. When I went down to visit them, I fell in love with the area.

I stuck it out a couple of years in that New York hospital so I wouldn't have to take a pay cut when I switched jobs. Then I went back down to Dunedin and walked into their medical center and asked if they had a job in the oncology unit there. The woman who interviewed me was the person I had replaced in New York. That was so bizarre, and we just sat and talked about Staten Island for the whole interview. "Of course you can work here," she said. "I know your hospital. I worked on your unit. You replaced me." She hired me on the spot, and I stayed there for two years.

There was an outpatient radiation/chemotherapy center across the street from the hospital, and one of the medical oncologists who worked there was from New York, too. Sometimes it felt like half the Empire State had moved to Florida to get warm. He had been a researcher, and he wasn't the easiest guy to get along with. His nurse was leaving, and she called to ask me if I would take her position, and I said, "No."

She said, "Why?"

"I don't like him. Plus, I'm working the 3 to 11 shift, and I've made a lot of friends. I'm having a good time."

"You need to take this position. Let me take you to lunch."

During lunch, she talked me into meeting with him.

In his office, the doctor didn't pull any punches: "I want you to come and work for me." He was one of these guys that you'd call and he'd hang up the phone on you. I'd always have to call him back and say, "Hey, look, this is your patient. I'm taking care of him. Tell me what you want me to do. Can I do this?" And he'd say, "Yeah, okay." He just liked that I would call him back and give him a hard time.

So I said, "First of all, I don't like you."

"Tell me what salary you want," he said.

I work 3:00 to 11:00, I thought. *I'll tell him what I make for working that shift, and he'll never go for it, and then I won't have to worry about it.* So I told him what I made, and he said, "I'll give you a dollar more an hour than that." So I took the job and stayed with him for eleven years. He really was very nice. He just acted badly because he thought he'd get more attention if he was cranky with people. He was a brilliant man – a researcher who had turned medical oncologist – and I learned a lot from him, too. I got to do chemo, and I got to do radiation. I worked with all the patients, and it was a great experience. Finally, he told me that I had to quit ruining his reputation by telling people how nice he was.

After eleven years with that doctor, I moved to Old Town, Florida, which is where I live now. I work at North Florida Regional Medical Center, but what I'd eventually like to do when I retire is to teach. I thought, *Well, if that's what I want, I really need to go back to school.* My mentor here has her master's degree, and she's an advanced registered nurse practitioner. She is our cancer program coordinator at the hospital, but she also sees patients, writes prescriptions, and goes out into the community and teaches. She helped me through my bachelor's degree, and recently she's been pushing me: "You need to go back. You just need to get your master's." So I'm studying now for my MSN in education, and eventually I know I'll look for teaching jobs.

Early in 2000, my thyroid cancer returned. I had remarried after I first moved to Florida, and a month after my treatment was successful, my husband got sick with his own cancer, and he didn't do very well. They cured his cancer, but his stomach flipped and he couldn't absorb any nourishment. His doctor advised him to go into hospice, and I said, "Wait a minute. I have an idea," and the doctor just stared at me.

"You say his cancer's cured, but you can't get his stomach to work. So let's just take it out. It's only a reservoir."

"He could die on the table," the doctor said.

"Well, you told me to put him in hospice. Why not try it? If he dies on the table, at least we gave him a chance."

Until last summer, I was Clinical Coordinator of the Oncology Unit at North Florida Regional Medical Center in Gainesville, and I had worked hand-in-hand with the doctors there. I wasn't intimidated by them. So telling my husband to go into hospice before we had tried all other options made no sense to me. Don't tell me you've cured something and then say he should just go and wait to die. So I got all the doctors together and said, "This is what I think we should do," and they agreed. They pumped his nutritional status up, did the surgery, and he came through with flying colors.

He has problems eating, of course, same as people who have had a gastric bypass. He doesn't have an esophagus either, so food goes directly into his small intestine. They did what they call a pull-up, where they stretch part of the stomach and make an esophagus out of that. Because the stomach acids can't break down the food, it goes into the intestine at a larger size. There are certain foods that he can't eat, like beef, which is hard to digest. But twelve years later, my husband is still with me.

Last August I changed jobs. The continuing challenge of coordinating seventy nurses with seventy different personalities finally became overwhelming. Plus, I was getting further and further away from patient care and felt it was time for a change. Now I'm a staff nurse on the night shift, and I'm remembering again how much I enjoy interacting with patients and staff.

Nursing, to me, means you can give back to people. You can make it easier for them to go through a really tough time. And if you can do that, it makes you feel good. When people find out I work in an oncology unit, they always say, "How can you work there? It's so depressing." I tell them, "Think of it this way: For me, the two most important times in your life are when you're born and when you die. When you're born, your family is happy and excited. When you're dying, don't you want your family to remember that it was peaceful? That's how I think of it, and I try to help that happen."

DR. AARON JUDKINS

I worked in a Level II trauma center in Fort Worth, Texas, for six years before I became an RN in 1998. But I wanted to be a flight nurse. I transferred to an ER because I wanted to gain additional experience in emergency nursing, and then I went back to school to become a licensed paramedic, as required by the Texas Department of Health. I gained the flight experience I needed by volunteering with Mercy Med Flight. I obtained my BSN with summa cum laude honors in 2007, and I hold a master of arts in biblical studies and a Ph.D. in biblical archeology.

As I tell nursing students, putting on that flight suit is a double-edged sword, and here's why: when people look at you, they only see the glory side of what you do; they don't experience the trauma side that is a big part of the job. They don't hold life-and-death decisions in their hands. Not only do you have the risk associated just with simply being in a machine that flies, putting your life in the hands of a pilot and a mechanic whom you hope are on their game that day, but you have multiple responsibilities. It's exciting, but it's also a very stressful environment.

You have to love it. You have to have a passion for it. But there are times when you get one of those terrible calls you hoped you'd never have to handle. It may be a complete third-degree burn; it may be a two-year-old in a traumatic full arrest. But let me tell you, when those calls come, you have to be ready for them, and you're never really ready for them. You can train, you can prepare, and you can do all those things that you're required to do, but when it happens, you never know how you're going to respond.

You have to make medical decisions on behalf of the doctor who is your coordinator. You actually function not only under your license, but you're functioning under his or her license as well. You can be connected by radio to that doctor, but you also have an A to Z protocol that gives you the authority to make most of those decisions. If you do have to call in, it's because there's a grey area somewhere. But you're still fully responsible.

I remember, we had a new flight nurse that came on, and she was solid. She knew her stuff. The very first day she went on duty, there was a pediatric double drowning at one of the area lakes. Both of those kids died, and she was finished. She didn't even ride back in the helicopter.

She got a ride back on one of the fire trucks. She said, "I'm done. I can't do this." Sometimes those things happen. It's a calling, I guess you could say. Either you have it or you don't. Most people can't understand the things you go through.

Nurses do experience some of those things in a hospital setting, but pre-hospital is a different story. You're in uncontrolled settings, like out in a pasture dealing with a farmer who's had his arm ripped off by some kind of a machine. You're not in the hospital. You don't have bright lights and sterile fields. You don't have a doctor right there. You're in the middle of an interstate; you're in a ditch; you're upside down in a car, trying to intubate someone to keep their airway open so the firefighters can cut him out. It's crazy stuff sometimes.

Back in 1989, when I graduated from Shamrock High School in Shamrock, Texas, I had no idea I'd end up being a nurse in a helicopter. I wasn't really sure what I wanted to do. I was working in a little market, sacking groceries. Now back then, I was getting $3.25 an hour. I had a friend who had gone to high school with me, and he had moved to Amarillo, where he was going to college. He called me up one day and said, "Man, I'm working at this nursing home, and I'm making five dollars an hour."

And I said, "What, are you kidding me? Five dollars an hour?"

"No, I'm not kidding," he said. "All you've got to do is learn how to take blood pressures and fill pitchers full of ice water for people – just do general things for them."

"Five dollars an hour sounds pretty good," I said.

So I moved out to Amarillo. I went to work at the nursing home with my friend, and I started to take some general courses at the community college there, too. I got a real behind-the-scenes view of nursing at that place. Of course, it was long-term care, but I realized that nursing might be a good avenue for me because it presented a whole variety of different possibilities.

Now, I didn't want to stay in long-term care, but I did want to prepare for nursing school. Trying to get through chemistry, and anatomy and physiology, I thought, *Man, these are hard classes. Microbiology? There's no way I'm going to be able to get through nursing school.* But I hung in there and passed all those classes, and I graduated from Amarillo College in 1991.

In Texas, they have LVNs – licensed vocational nurses – and that's what I went for. I had pretty much decided that nursing was the field that would work best for me as a career. After I graduated from LVN school in Arlington, Texas, I went through an ICU rotation, and that really opened my eyes. It was such a different environment, and I wanted to work there. But critical care at that time was an RN-based specialty. I was working at John Peter Smith Hospital, which was a Level II trauma center in Fort Worth. That's a teaching hospital, and I knew I could get all my experience there. They used to say that six months working in a Level II trauma center equals a year anywhere else.

So I started off in the telemetry unit, and that gave me a foundation for learning advanced cardiac life support. We monitored people – that was the nature of our unit. We did have cardiac patients who would come in, and I learned the fundamentals of critical care at the very basic level. I had to read rhythms and learn how to treat them, and I stayed there for three years.

The critical care unit at John Peter Smith was RN-based as well, but they did take one exceptional LVN on the day shift and one on the night shift. And after working the three years in the telemetry unit and getting my fundamentals there, an opening in the ICU came up, and I was accepted. Of course, I had a good foundation. I knew medications. I knew pharmacology. I knew a lot about chronic diseases from working initially as a nurse-tech in the nursing home.

But that critical care unit was the opposite end of the spectrum from the nursing home. First of all, the patients varied in age. Secondly, in the critical care unit, people were having heart attacks, and there was trauma all the time. But even though they were acutely ill, most of the patients got better and were discharged. I was able to see positive results as I went through and treated them, and I liked the fact that I could make decisions and really affect the outcomes in that setting. I was young. I was gung-ho. I loved the adrenaline rush, and critical care really gave me that. Things can turn on a dime, and you're right there.

When I precept students, I tell them, "There are nurses who work in critical care, and then there are critical-care nurses, and there's a vast difference between them." With the critical care nurses, you could tell they had a foundation, a specialty – they weren't just nurses. They functioned autonomously. They didn't have to rely on a panel to make a decision. They made their decisions based on either objective, clinical data that they were receiving or on subjective, observed phenomena – meaning specific things they observed that made a difference. Something that appears to be minor on the surface may be the key that signals a profound underlying problem. Critical-care nurses are able to discover those particular things that make a difference in patient outcomes. To be a critical-care nurse, you have to take ownership, because there are life-and-death decisions that have to be made.

There are nurses who work in critical care who aren't quite up to that level yet. No one walks in fully accomplished – that takes experience. It takes someone to mentor you. It takes continual education to get you to that point. Now some people are better than others: they catch on faster; they're quicker learners. But most nurses, when they come into the ICU, it's a new thing for them. They have to work their way up to that level. When they get there, though, you can definitely tell the ones who are making that difference.

In 1998, after I earned my associate's degree in nursing, I took my boards and got my RN. That opened up a whole new range of work settings for me. By that time, I had worked for six years as a critical-care nurse, and I decided my next goal was to become a flight nurse. I had seen one of the helicopter-based programs operating around Dallas-Fort Worth. I was stopped in traffic by a serious accident, and I saw one come in and land on the highway. I watched as they treated the patient, loaded him up, and flew off, and I thought, *That's what I want to do. I've got the training, as far as the critical care aspect, and I know I can do that.*

The immediate attraction was that it was outside the hospital setting. You could be totally independent because you're considered pre-hospital. It's more in emergency services, and I grew up watching *MASH* and *Emergency* and all those early-'70s rescue shows on TV. They were what inspired me. I wouldn't be stuck in a building twelve hours a day.

As much as I loved critical care, I had done that, and I wanted to take my career to the next level.

Well, there's no flight nurse school, per se. So how do you become one? I just went around and talked to different people and asked for their recommendations. "You probably need to go work in the ER," a bunch of them told me. "You need to get out of critical care. You've got that. You need to get your certifications."

So I transferred from critical care to the emergency room, which was a lot different. In critical care, you have to be detail-oriented, and you're working in a structured setting. The ER is totally the opposite: not very structured, and you've always got a variety of patients coming in – very fast-paced. You're not writing pages of notes, the way you are in ICU, where sometimes you can take your time doing some of those things. In the ER, it's quick, and I had to learn how to function in that setting. On top of that, I had to go back to school again. The Texas Department of Health requires flight nurses to be certified on the helicopter, so I went back to school in 1999 to get my paramedic training, and I became a licensed paramedic that year.

Then I got a chance to volunteer for Mercy Med Flight, which was founded by a man named Ken McAlear. He was the personal pilot for Tom Landry, former head coach of the Dallas Cowboys. When Tom Landry got cancer, Ken McAlear would fly him to Houston, to the M.D. Anderson Cancer Center, for his treatments. Ken started Mercy Med Flight as a charitable service after that. It's no longer in existence, but it was a really great service. Our patients were people who had long-term care conditions. Whatever their needs were, Ken didn't charge to transport them.

We took those missions on advance notice. They were scheduled, so I would know on a particular day that we would fly a certain mission. They would call and say, "We have a mission to so and so on this day. Can you accept it?" And nine times out of ten, I would. I'd work twelve-hour night shifts in the ER, and then I'd get off at 7 A.M, and I'd have a thirty-five-minute drive into Fort Worth.

My partner, Jeff, and I would pre-flight the aircraft about 7:45 a.m., and at 8:00 a.m. sharp, we were on the runway taking off. Back in those days, I was in my late twenties, and I didn't sleep that much. I'd work all night and then I'd fly all day. Then I'd go to sleep for a couple of hours before my ER shift started. On some of those missions, though, we were able to spend the night. If it was a long mission, like over to California, we would fly over and stay the night and fly back home the next day. Most of the time, they were same-day turnarounds.

With Mercy, I flew in a 421 Golden Eagle Cessna aircraft, a turboprop twin engine. That basically gave me the flight experience I needed, even though it was fixed-wing. Back in those days, I volunteered probably 50 percent of my time. Now this was before I had kids. But after Mercy shut its doors, I got a job on the rotor-wing helicopter, which was a 911 service. We got toned out, like firefighters. It's a very sudden change of your schedule, and you have to be ready to go. The first service that I flew with was Critical Air, but that company was sold. Then I went over and flew with PHI (Petroleum Helicopters, Inc.).

Being a nurse in an aircraft is totally different, and you have to learn to function in that setting. It's cold. There's a lot of noise and vibration that make it hard to hear. You have to rely on visual alarms more than audible alarms, so you really have to watch the monitor lights. There's not a lot of space to move around in. You have to be aware of physiological changes at altitude, so I had to learn and study all those changes that can occur.

And then you have to learn how to deal with the losses. I had this one, solid week of pediatric traumas. When I got those, it was a whole different ball game. For some people, it might not be, but for me, pediatrics was my Achilles heel. I always said to myself, *Okay, I haven't dealt with my first pediatric death yet. If one comes up, I'm just going to have to deal with it.* But, you know, I didn't have just one pediatric death: I had an entire week of them.

It started off with a mass casualty incident on Interstate 35. We got up in the air and called in. There was one firefighter who was in radio communication with us, and we could tell from his voice when he yelled, "MASS CASUALTY," into the radio. There were very few people on scene when we went in. I think maybe the highway patrol and some construction crews were there, but we could tell it was going to be bad as soon as we landed.

It was a van, full of a family coming back from Mexico. The dad had fallen asleep at the wheel. When it rolled, two of the kids were ejected. One of them, a four-year-old, was thrown into the ditch, and one was a ten-year-old, also in the ditch but the van had rolled on top of him. So my partner and I split up.

There was one strange detail. When we landed, all I can remember tortillas all over the highway. That's ingrained in my memory. I saw them and I thought, *Why are all these tortillas on the highway? They're just all over the place.* Then I connected the dots. They were coming back from Mexico and had packages of food in the car and the tortillas got thrown all over the highway when the van rolled. I just remember stepping over all the scattered tortillas and having this terrible feeling in the pit of my stomach.

So the ten-year-old who was under the van, we couldn't get him out. He was still conscious, but he didn't know English. There was a firefighter with him. I know a little medical Spanish, and I asked him if he was hurting. He said he wasn't. That was a bad sign.

At that point, I took his hand and held it. I don't think he understood me, but sometimes communication isn't verbal. To be a good nurse, you have to know your stuff, act independently, and meet the needs of your patient. Sometimes that means simply holding a child's hand.

I like the saying I heard one time: "It takes a nurse to save your life." Yes, doctors are there, and they have their purpose. They initiate the treatments and the orders and everything but, in reality, it takes a nurse to save your life, because the nurse is the one there with you. Where the doctors are always coming and going, the nurse is there. The nurses are the quiet heroes, and especially the emergency nurses. It's the helicopter flight nurses who are the quiet heroes. It's the hospice nurses who hold someone's hand in the last moments before death who are the quiet heroes. That's the compassion of nursing. If you don't have that ability to be compassionate, you shouldn't be in nursing.

So I just grabbed his hand and held it. Even though I couldn't talk to him, I looked him in the eyes, and I took my other hand and I rubbed his head. I told him he was going to be okay. Of course, I don't know if he understood that. But I gave him the best reassurance and compassion that I could give anyone. We called in a second helicopter to get him out once they got him extricated from the van. But both of those kids ended up dying.

Then the very next day, I had a nine-year-old girl who was in a go-kart that didn't have a roll bar in the front. It was just an open go-kart. She was going down a little hill on a residential street near where she lived and she couldn't stop. Either she didn't know how to brake or she didn't brake in time, but she ran up underneath a parked truck, and it crushed her chest.

When we got to her, she was extremely pale. Her little tummy was hard as a rock, and she wasn't saying anything. I asked her, "Honey, are you hurting," and she didn't answer me. She shook her head no. I knew that was it. She wasn't screaming, and she wasn't crying. When I saw her pasty color and I realized she was just quiet, I scooped her up and ran with her to the helicopter. I knew that she probably wasn't going to make it.

We didn't have room to take her mom in the helicopter with us, but I had her come alongside with me. Right before we loaded her daughter, I gave the mom thirty seconds. I told her, "Mom, you've got thirty seconds with your daughter and then we're going to have to leave. But you should come to the hospital." I didn't know for sure that was the last time her mother was going to see her alive, but something told me, *Let this mother hold her child's hand just for a few seconds.* Normally, I should have immediately loaded the patient in and we should have taken off. So that last thirty seconds that mother got with her was crucial, I think, and I'm so glad I made that decision to let her do that.

That week was more than hard for me. My son had been born about a year and a half earlier, and when I called home, I was really struggling. I had been in the nursing field at that time for about fifteen years, and I had seen hundreds of people die. I had saved probably hundreds of people, too, but I had also seen a lot of people die, so death wasn't a new thing for me. But those pediatric deaths hit me especially hard.

So I called home at the end of the shift. It was late, and it was out of character for me to call late, and my wife said, "What are you doing?" And I said, "Take the phone and go put it by my son's head. Let me hear him. Just put it by his mouth and let me hear him breathing for a minute." So she did, and then she got back on the phone. I told her what had happened, and that really gave me a calming measure.

I had a flight paramedic who had been in the business for a long time, and he gave me some really good advice. He said, "Aaron, we didn't put them in that situation. We're there to help them the best way we know how. We do all we can do, but sometimes that's not enough." Then he said something I'll never forget: "Aaron, here's something that has helped me in the past, and I think it will help you. Rule #1 is that people die. Rule #2 is that you can't change Rule #1." And I thought, *You know what? I'm going to take that. We're not here to be miracle workers. We're here to give them the best chance at life that we can with our training. And then the rest is up to God.*

I stopped flying a little while after that. Our company's sister helicopter went down in Arizona one night, and some of the crew were killed. We got the call around midnight, right after I had returned from a flight. *Thanks for that call,* I thought. *I've got to go to bed now. I've got another six hours on duty and I haven't slept a minute. We may get another flight, and now I've got this in my head, too.*

Soon after that, I had a friend who was a year ahead of me in high school, who had also become a flight nurse, and she died. She worked for the Amarillo service helicopter, and they took a night call where the weather moved in, with fog. They took a pediatric patient up and then they hit a wire and it killed all of them. EMS and helicopters and pre-hospital – that's a pretty tight world: people learn what's going on in that world within hours, usually. So my wife heard about both of those accidents. To calm her fears about it, I decided to ground myself until our son got a little older, and I went back to work at the hospital in 2005.

Let me tell you, nursing is sometimes a thankless job. You can save people all day long. You can do everything possible, but nine times out of ten, it's a thankless job at the end of the day. You go home and you're stressed. You've worked twelve hours on your feet. You've barely had time to eat, and hardly had the time to go to the bathroom. You go home, go to sleep, then get back up and do it again. You're not in it for the glory, and you're not in it for the money. You have to have a passion for working with people to do this job.

But like it or not, I've got that passion, and now I'm back flying with AeroCare Medical Transport team in Arizona as a flight nurse servicing the Navajo Nation. We provide fixed-wing air medical transport to the rural Four Corners Region of the United States, as well as in Tulsa, Oklahoma, where AeroCare is headquartered. I have had some really blessed times, taking care of people whom I never would have been able to take care of in my life, and I get to know them on some occasions. It's not for everyone, but it's something that I truly enjoy. And by the way, here's the full set of my rules:

Aaron's Top 10 List of Nursing Rules

1. People die.
2. You can't change Rule #1.
3. What can go wrong, will go wrong (Murphy's Law).
4. When in doubt, ACT.
5. If you're not sure, look it up.
6. Don't treat the monitor – treat the patient.
7. If you think you should call the doctor, you probably should.
8. Always notify the doctor for a change in patient's condition &/ or vital signs.
9. If you didn't document it, it didn't happen.
10. Treat others as you would want to be treated.

NICOLE SHOUNDER

In 1995, when I left the Air Force, I did agency nursing and covered a large segment of the field. I worked as a nurse in an adult, close-custody medium-security prison, and on a bone-marrow transplant unit at Fred Hutchinson Cancer Research Center. I was part of the FEMA National Disaster Medical System and deployed to Houston after Hurricane Alison, and to Louisiana after Hurricanes Rita and Katrina. I began my maritime nursing career on the USNS Impeccable, *a submarine-surveillance ship operated by Maersk Line Limited. Then I worked on ships that supported the ships chasing pirates in the Gulf of Aden and off the coast of Somalia. Currently, I am serving on the USS* Ponce.

Traveling has been in my blood from the beginning, and what a long, strange trip it's been. My dad was in the Air Force, and my mom worked civil service jobs on the bases where my dad was stationed. We bounced around from the late '50s, when I was born, until the mid-'70s. There were two bases in Alaska, one in Texas, and another in Oklahoma. We spent a good long time in Dover, Delaware, and then my dad retired to Lancaster, Pennsylvania.

Living near Dover Air Force Base in the early '70s was very poignant for me. I grew up seeing the stacks and stacks of what I called the aluminum suitcases – the flight coffins coming back from the war in Vietnam. At the time, I thought, *If that's the number of people who are dying, my God, how many people are being hurt and wounded?* So I decided I wanted to be a combat paramedic. That way I could rescue soldiers before they died. Then I realized how short a medic's life span would be and I thought, *No, maybe I could do more elsewhere if I lived longer.*

In Lancaster, I joined the Mannheim VFW volunteer ambulance association, and I was an EMT before I graduated from Mannheim Central High School in 1977. The next year, I went into the Air Force and did basic and medical training in Texas. I was assigned first to Loring Air Force Base, Strategic Air Command, in northern Maine. Being a gung-ho guy in my former life, before my operation, I had originally planned to try for the males-only Air Force Pararescue program. But my dad had seen too many of his friends not return from the war, and he put the old kibosh on that idea. So I transferred to Wichita Falls, Texas, and studied to become an independent duty medical technician, an IDMT, which is like a mobile hospital in a single human package.

We learned how to handle sick call, treat patients, administer immunizations, and even do minor dental work. IDMT school was where the nursing seed in me got cultivated.

Eventually I was selected for a special-duty assignment with the Air Force Combat Survival School, and I moved up to Washington State for that. I went through SERE training – that's survival and evasion, resistance and escape – at Fairchild Air Force Base near Spokane. I worked directly with the survival instructors there, learning how to use a parachute and live off the land, as well as acquiring a long list of other skills that would satisfy any adrenaline junkie in the country.

However, the reduction-in-force writing was on the wall in the military, and I wanted to get a nursing degree while I still had financial support. At that point, I had thirteen years of military education and training under my belt, and that earned me a lot of credit transfer when I enrolled in a distance education program. During my six months of transitional assistance as a civilian, I completed all the course work for my associate's degree in nursing, and I passed my clinicals in San Diego.

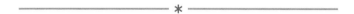

Before my nursing license came through, I was working as a medical assistant in the outpatient cancer unit at St. Joseph's Hospital in Tacoma, Washington. Right about that time, my family situation was pretty tenuous. I was in the final stages of determining whether or not I would go through transition for my gender issues. The nurses I worked with at St. Joe's were very understanding and appreciative of my skills and desire to work. We had all gotten to know each other pretty well, and they realized that things were approaching a real breaking point with me and my family. One day, the Chief Nurse there pulled me off to the side and said, "Look, we value who and what you are. We want you to stay working here, but we need you to make a decision rather than waffling. It's becoming pretty tense for some of the nurses."

Basically, she was saying she wanted me to take a couple of months off on the employee assistance program and figure out what I needed to do. "If you can't, and if there isn't any change," she said, "I'm probably going to have to let you go. And by the way, if you do value what people think, nine out of the twelve nurses here actually like Nicole better than they like Nick."

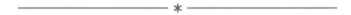

After my reassignment surgery, and with my nursing license in hand, I started working for an agency. Supposedly, there was a nursing glut at that time, in the late '90s, so I couldn't get hired full time as an RN at hospitals where I had worked as a medical assistant before. However, since I had been an IDMT in the Air Force and knew emergency medicine, and because I had my ACLS certification already, I was immediately qualified through the agency for work in telemetry step-down units and, a little later, in ICUs. Literally, I would jump from a long-term care environment where I was replacing a floor nurse – handing out meds, doing treatments, and reviewing Medicare care plans on one day – to a slot filling in for a vacationing nurse in a neuro-transplant ICU.

I had an agreement with my agency boss, the scheduler: I was his to use and abuse in whatever capacity he needed for the first forty hours a week, and then from there I would start to be selective about where I went for overtime. I was driving up and down I-5, eighty miles or more at a crack, to different facilities, and the constant commuting wasn't easy. But what made me especially happy was that I was being paid more to work per diem as a temp than I would have made as regular staff. Finally, I did get hired for a longer stretch at the Fred Hutchinson Cancer Research Center as a clinical research nurse on the inpatient unit. They had experienced an unexpected surge in ICU patients and needed to bring in a handful of nurses on a long-term basis.

The one thing that really stands out for me about my time at the Fred Hutchinson Center was how it changed the way I viewed the process of dying. Before that job, I would say I saw my role as primarily helping people to get healthy and move ahead with their lives. When someone had a terminal diagnosis, though, that role had to change. In my time there, I came to understand the importance of hospice and palliative

THE CALL OF NURSING

care: *How could I offer patients and their families a calm, solid closure to life? How could I help them achieve a good death?*

There was one particular situation I remember where a daughter had to make a decision about stopping advanced life support for her father. Transplant complications had overwhelmed his body. The doctor had explained the options to her and estimated a 30 percent chance of survival with even the most radical procedure. That 30 percent had swelled to 90 percent in her mind, though, because she needed to believe that. *How could I help her understand the reality of her father's situation, and how could I establish the necessary rapport?*

It sounds impersonal to discuss the nuts and bolts of establishing rapport with a family member – of essentially exercising compassion when you deliver difficult information to her. That should be instinctive and easy, right? But when you hardly know someone, or when you have to perform that compassionate task several times a day, the nuts and bolts become important. In one sense, there's the mechanical side: try to get into a position where you're physically lower than the person to whom you're speaking, so they're looking down at you rather than up. Speak to them at close range, not from across a desk. Make sure they can reach out to you if they need physical contact. Those kinds of strategies.

But the mechanical side doesn't touch a person's heart or soul. If what you say in that moment isn't heartfelt and human and genuine, it will do more harm than good. I did know that her father had fought in Vietnam, so I told her I was sure he could soldier on no matter what. He would continue to carry the load for his family without any concern for himself, just as he had done at his job and in supporting his family all those years. But there would come a point when his pack would get too heavy, and that he was very close to that point.

Acting like a drill instructor, yelling, "You've got to get back up, and you've got to keep going," wasn't going to make his pack any lighter or his legs any stronger. At some point, she would have to respect the fact that her father had given all that he could give. I told her that, with technology, we could keep his body going for quite a while. Even though there was a time when he might have told her, "Honey, do everything you can. I have to be there for you," she had to help him stop. That was hard for her, but she understood, and thanked me.

There is a toll that compassion exacts from nurses, though. The more you let yourself be vulnerable, the closer you can come to burning out, because those intense emotions haunt you. The more you empathize, in my experience, the more oppressive it can become. After a few months there, I realized I had to get out of the cancer center.

About that time, I learned about the volunteer program that FEMA and the National Disaster Medical System had in place. After 9/11, and in response to the anthrax scare that swept through the nation, there was a push to prepare federal disaster-response teams for similar biological emergencies, and the smallpox inoculation program was reinstated. Disaster teams were supposed to be inoculated so they could respond in the event of an emergency. I volunteered, and the people at Fred Hutchinson Center freaked out, because they had to guarantee their patients that there was zero chance of transmission of smallpox.

I was already feeling a little burned out from my months of dealing with terminal patients, so when the Nursing Director at the Cancer Center asked me if I would forego the shot and ascribe to what she called "a higher philosophy of life and care," I answered, "I certainly will. I'm transferring to the ER and working down there so I can get this inoculation and be able to respond if our nation experiences a crisis."

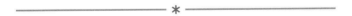

For four years in that emergency department, I worked six twelve-hour night shifts for a week and then had the following week off. That was enough for a while. Then I had a brief stint working as a prison nurse. I lasted until my last day of probation, when they let me go. It wasn't the gender issue, and they loved the work I did. They felt the fit wasn't right.

Part of my training at the Air Force Survival School had involved working in a fake prisoner of war camp, where we taught people how to manipulate guards. So at the prison, if I were called to a cell because someone was supposedly puking his guts out and needed IV fluids or an injection to settle them down, I'd assess the situation and usually say, "Nope, you're not really puking. I see lots of tissue in the garbage can, I see lots of phlegm, but I don't smell anything. That's page 13 out of the manipulation manual. Good try, though."

The Nursing Director of the prison told me she was really sorry to let me go. If I put in a request for a reference to any place but another corrections facility, she would make sure it was a glowing, positive reference. "Don't go back to prison care," she said. I asked her why, and she said, "Honestly, Nicole, you make a better prison guard than you do a nurse. Everyone said that if there was a riot on the floor, they'd want you on shift when it happens." A year or so after I left there, sure enough, there was a riot in the yard, and a couple of people were seriously injured.

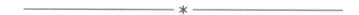

After I volunteered at The St. Charles Parish Hospital in Louisiana with the Washington One Disaster Medical Assistance Team during Katrina and Rita, you'd think I would have been sick of water. But that's when I applied for my Merchant Marine documents, in 2006, to be a professional nurse, hospital corpsman, and junior assistant purser, entry level. Boating had been my hobby for several years at that point, and I had even volunteered with the Coast Guard Auxiliary.

During one of my classes with them, I was getting my boat squared away when a guy with a heavy Scottish accent approached me and said he heard I was a nurse who worked in an emergency department. "If you like being on the water, I've got a boat," he said. "It's *The Northern Eagle*, and we go trawler processor factory fishing in the Bering Sea. I think you'd be a good fit."

"That's nice," I said, "but I don't know you." People ran over afterwards and told me, "That was Captain Sandy Ritchie. He runs one of the biggest fishing trawlers out of Seattle, and he just offered you a job. Folks line up around the block to work on that ship." I looked it up on Google and sure enough, it was over four hundred feet long and had a crew of two hundred. That's when I applied for Merchant Marine documents. But before they arrived, Captain Ritchie called to say they were shipping out. He'd try me in six months.

In the meantime, I had to get trained all over again. I worked in the ER during the week and flew to San Diego every weekend for a month and a half, getting all my credentials recertified from the Independent Duty side. On top of that, I had to revalidate what I needed for Merchant Marine Emergency Medical certification. It started with emergency safety stuff, from firefighting to helicopter crash rescue to damage control for a hole in the side of the ship, but it also included recertifying in pest control, food inspection, food facility inspection, domestic and tropical diseases – even how to identify malaria on a microscope slide.

When my papers finally arrived, I went looking for a maritime job. I ended up on the 280-foot USNS *Impeccable*, an ocean surveillance ship that was operated by the Maersk Lines. It functioned as a giant floating sonar marker. There were forty-five crew members on board who, for months at a time, would need medical and dental care. The *Impeccable* was where I got to renew the dental skills I had learned in IDMT school.

For instance, one active duty sailor was hooking up some equipment over the moon pool – the hole in the ship that equipment was lowered through – and the seas were kind of rough that day. The block and tackle slipped and caught him in the face. Fortunately, he jerked back enough so it only nailed his lip and chipped the front of his tooth off. He wasn't bleeding too much. Well, it was my first dental job since training, but I didn't tell him that. I numbed the front of his face and then inspected all his other teeth for damage. I was able to fill and shape it to match the unbroken tooth beside it, and it held up okay for the two weeks it took us to reach port. It wasn't terribly dramatic, but it was a success.

Jobs with the Maersk lines were six months on and six months off, so pretty soon I needed a second maritime job. I called Captain Ritchie and said, "I'm still interested in learning the position," and it was the right timing. I went out with *The Northern Eagle* for six months in the Bering Sea. We literally went up to St. Mary's, where they film *The Deadliest*

Catch. It was a wild trip, and there was good money in it. And when we returned to Seattle, I went back to the *Impeccable*.

———————————— ✳ ————————————

Being out on the sea, you have to take joy and solace in what are minor triumphs along the way. I had a forty-eight-year-old guy who stroked out on me in the middle of the Red Sea, and I had to stabilize him until we could get him off the ship. I'm proud to say that he was stabilized by early recognition, even though a lot of people thought he was faking it. That happened on the USNS *Robert E. Peary*, the fourth Navy ship named for the Arctic explorer, and one of Military Sealift Command's fourteen dry cargo/ammunition ships. It's a monster, almost 700 feet long, with a crew of 170, and it gave me my first voyage off the coast of Somalia and up into the Persian Gulf and the Gulf of Aden. With that one I came up with the phrase "I chase ships that chase pirates." We would bring the destroyers the food, fuel, and supplies they needed to stay on station and continue their anti-piracy missions.

I was the only medical officer on board, and I was literally with the guy when his stroke started. I watched the minor paralysis begin in his face. As I said in my notes to the doctor, "I watched his face melt right before my eyes." Immediately I laid him down flat and we put him into a Stokes basket. Eight people carried him down four flights of stairs to the sick bay, and I basically commenced running around with my hair on fire: putting in a Foley catheter, starting an IV, getting oxygen going, monitoring the stroke's progress as best I could, contacting people on the telephone, and having people call for a helicopter with the ship's satellite radio.

Finally, we got him medevacked off the boat. He went to a foreign national hospital in the United Arab Emirates for a month, where it was validated that he had suffered two strokes. He was further stabilized there and then was flown back to the United States. After some rehabilitation, he actually came back to a ship I was on. He was grateful and boasted to the crew about how capable I was. It was heartwarming, of course, but I was just apprehensive that he'd have another stroke.

Currently, I'm on the USS *Ponce*. Last year, this ship was reconfigured to support mine countermeasure operations and act as a mission support vessel for Fifth Fleet operations. We're in the Persian Gulf, serving as the Pentagon's first floating base for military operations or humanitarian assistance. I'm the Medical Service Officer on board but, for a change, I have a coworker, a Navy Independent Duty Corpsman. Basically, I'm doing for this crew what I've done for the crews of the other ships. I'm kind of like a Lego. I do the same job no matter where I go and what I'm responsible for. Whatever the ship does as its mission is the thing that changes and adds flavor to the quality of my life.

———————————— * ————————————

Let me share strategies that I passed on to student nurses when I was working the floor as an agency nurse. Get to thinking things through graphically in your mind. There are a lot of television shows, like *CSI* and *NOVA* and others, where they show you what's happening physiologically. Either it's the trauma – a bullet tearing through tissue, severing this or damaging that or lodging somewhere – or in some shows where they might be talking about snakebites and the neurotoxins being transmitted, they'll show you graphically, at the cellular level, what's going on. You can learn a mental technique from those shows. When you do an assessment, imagine all the body systems at one time to get a total picture of what is happening to an individual. You can actually start to predict how some things are going to evolve because you can see them, inside your mind, beginning to happen.

Secondly, just because the organization that you work for expects problem-oriented nursing assessments, there's no reason that you can't do a very rapid nursing assessment in two solid minutes with a patient, covering all the body systems. You can get them to go through the basics pretty quickly: cranio-facial, squint your eyes, move your jaw, stick your tongue out, shrug your shoulders, grab my hands. Get the basics of the cranials and the peripherals out of the way first.

Then listen to the lungs, heart, and stomach. From there, finish up with the skin assessment. By covering all these areas very quickly, you can not only cover the problem your patient is presenting but you can discover any number of other things. Basically, it would constitute what most people would call your intake assessment on a person. If you get used to doing that each time you start off with a patient, you may be one step ahead of where an illness might be heading. Once you develop your system, it will become second nature.

I have loved bringing nursing into a job which is traditionally an Independent Duty Corpsman role. I try to bring a holistic approach to the health care I provide, and I attempt to integrate better preventive medicine into the maritime culture. I work with people to help them understand what they need to do to stay healthy, and how they can safeguard themselves in isolated, remote environments. I'm a living example that this is a job that you can take literally around the world and adapt to perform a duty that people genuinely need.

TAMMY WARREN

*I became a nurse as the result of my
experience as a combat medic assigned to
a female medical-surgical ward at Brooke
Army Medical Center in San Antonio, Texas.
I trained in the Army's Practical Nurse
Program, and I became the senior NCO in
charge of the Hematology/Oncology ward.
I served as the patient safety manager
at Munson Army Health Center on the
base at Fort Leavenworth, Kansas, before
I transitioned back to my current job at
Munson's Family Medicine Clinic.*

Leavenworth, Kansas, where I live and work, is famous for its prisons. We have the medium-security Leavenworth federal prison, the United States Disciplinary Barracks, which is the military's only maximum security prison, and the Midwest Joint Regional Correctional Facility, which opened in 2010. It's a pre-confinement facility. Many of the folks you may see on television who are awaiting confinement may be sitting right here in Leavenworth. A lot of them appear frequently on CNN.

Before I went back to the family medicine clinic, I was the patient safety manager at Munson Army Health Center, which is an ambulatory care facility on the Fort Leavenworth base. We're an outpatient facility only, and we perform orthopedic surgery, GYN surgery, ENT surgery, and general surgery. They're all same-day surgeries, and our patients go home by 4:30 or 5:00 p.m.

For that job, I delivered a lot of education to staff: there was a monthly newcomer's orientation where I explained about the program that we have here and how it's affiliated with the Army's Department of Defense Patient Safety Program, and I talked about the shared goals that we have in order to provide safe care for our patients. And I did a lot of tracers, or inspections. I went around observing people, and I encouraged them to follow our guidelines, which align with the National Patient Safety Goals established by The Joint Commission in 2003. Then I not only gave feedback to the command on how we could better meet those goals, but I also offered a presentation to staff about how all of us at Munson needed to be aware of those goals as well.

That sounds pretty dry, doesn't it? Why should we be concerned about patient safety goals? Here's a simple example: Because we're a military facility, a lot of folks think all they need is a military ID in order to come visit us. To be a beneficiary here, you require military ID. So some folks would think that's one of our two patient identifiers, when in fact it's not. Our two patient identifiers are a patient's full name and birthday. The military ID card is just a tool we use to make sure you're eligible for benefits. It may seem like a minor thing, but when we do that procedure, give that injection, or prescribe that medication, it's important to know we have the right patient. That's one of the goals.

Here's another seemingly small example: Are you on any medications? Do you always carry a list of them with you? You should, because in the event of an emergency, if you weren't able to speak, people could determine what you're taking. That way, you have a better chance of avoiding adverse drug interactions during treatment, and that could very well save your life.

Let me make it personal. My father takes cardiac medications. When he came to visit me recently, he was frequently dizzy. He was waiting to have a cardiac catheterization done to open up one of his stents, and he blamed the dizziness on that. It really was debilitating for him. So I convinced my mother to give me a list of all his medications. What I discovered was that his doctor had changed his meds, but my dad was still taking the meds he had gotten three months earlier. He's on a fixed budget, so he couldn't afford to waste money, and he decided to complete the old meds. Is that a problem? Yes, because there are lots of potentials when it comes to medications, and a drastic procedure in an ER can be the result. In fact, adverse medication events injure more patients than any other health care problem.

Another key concern with patient-safety goals is suicide. The Pentagon just announced that suicides in the military have reached epidemic proportions. During the last year, more soldiers died by killing themselves than died in combat. So it's essential that we identify those who might be in danger of harming themselves or others. Many of our returning soldiers suffer from PTSD, and they're at a pronounced risk for suicide, so we ask them a simple question at the start of every clinic appointment: "How are you feeling today?" or "Have you felt unhappy or depressed recently?" or even, simply, "How's it going?"

The response to one of those questions will lead you to other questions. An immediate red flag would go up if they just answered yes to a question about whether they were depressed, because most folks don't answer that question truthfully. If you ask people how they're doing, they'll say, "I'm doing okay." People don't often share how they truly feel.

The key is to convince our soldiers that we care about how they are on any given day. It's not a matter of asking – it's the way that we ask. It's observing them as they walk down our hallways. Are they walking with their heads down, dragging their feet, shoulders slumped over? If our staff members see someone who looks distraught, they should say something. If they happen to be coming back from lunch and walk past a patient who clearly is in need, they should stop and ask if they can help. We try to encourage and empower everyone to be fully aware of what's going on around them.

One of the key esprit de corps things that we try to do in the military is offer the greeting of the day. Whenever I first see you, I offer that, "Hello. How are you? Good morning." It's not about me. It's all about you. People will either make considered contact or they won't, and if they don't, that could be an indication something is wrong. You can change someone's day by simply giving them the greeting of the day.

In order to help us identify potential suicides, we have a program here called respect.mil. We have a physician who facilitates that program. Active-duty soldiers who are identified as being at risk can get one-on-one consultation with a nurse case manager. We try hard to identify those patients and to make sure they're okay, and we have resources in place for them.

I retired from the military in 2004, after twenty years. In some ways, I miss that life. I guess that's why I still work on an Army base. I enlisted when I was still in high school because I wanted to get away from my father. I ran cross-country and track. He didn't like my friends who were on the cross-country and track teams with me, and he said I couldn't see them. That didn't really make logical sense to me. My father's rules didn't coincide with what I believed or what I wanted for myself so, out of respect, I felt it was best to leave home.

I moved out in September, the start of my senior year, and I worked part time at Wendy's. I had an efficiency apartment that I paid for with my Wendy's salary. It was $186 a month – almost everything I made. I was lucky that my sister would bring me a bag of groceries and put it under my chair in Spanish class. Another friend gave me a block of Velveeta cheese. In Wendy's, the only thing they didn't recycle back then were the potatoes. They recycle them now. But back then they didn't, and sometimes there were leftover chicken filets, too. They didn't recycle those, at least not the fried ones. So when I had to close, I would get the baked potatoes, and sometimes I'd get lucky and someone would forget about a chicken, and I'd have that, too. There are an amazing number of ways that you can fix a baked potato, especially with a block of Velveeta cheese. When I think back, I really wasn't lacking anything: I had an apartment, and I had wheels. My bicycle got me to work, or to and from school. And I had hot-chocolate Tuesdays. Hot-chocolate Tuesdays meant that my grandmother would stop by and we would sit at my little table and we'd have hot chocolate and then she'd take me to school.

But I ran out of money by Christmas, so I joined the Army. I got permission to graduate early, and I finished up on January 31st. The recruiter took me down to the post office, and I took the exam. I had a choice of any job I wanted because I had scored high on the exam. I chose truck driver, which was a 64 Charlie back then. I thought, Well, my father's a truck driver, so I probably should be able to drive a rig, right? Not ever having even handled a rig or anything. Yeah, it's hereditary. I should be able to get it.

But on the way back from military entrance processing in Indianapolis, we got caught in a snowstorm and we did a couple of little doughnuts in the K car, and I was thinking, I really don't think I could handle a rig in this weather. So I was able to get my 64 Charlie changed to what was called 91 Bravo, which is a combat medical specialist. I actually went on active duty on Groundhog Day, and was sent to Fort Sam Houston, in San Antonio.

My father wouldn't sign for me to go into the military because I had defied him. He grew up in the era where he believed, "I'm the parent and you do as I say." And he was very private, too. I didn't know a lot about him. I didn't know how he was raised or his background. He never really communicated much of anything to me. However, after I turned eighteen and had enlisted, I found out that he had served in the Army and was stationed in Korea during the war there. As it turned out, we never really had a reason to sit down and discuss why things happened the way they happened. You just make decisions and move on, and you find a way to live with those decisions.

After I graduated from AIT, advanced individual training, I stayed in San Antonio. They needed a handful of women medics to stay and work at Brooke Army Medical Center. That was my first introduction to nursing. I worked on 42 E, which is a female surgical unit, and we had a head nurse whose name was Mrs. Traficante. We called her Mrs. T. She was about five feet eleven, and she was in her seventies. She had that little white cap that she wore on her head all the time, and a starched uniform, and shiny white shoes. She would make sure that we had all the patients bathed and their beds changed, on the day shift, before 10:00 a.m., before our first break. So everyone was just rushing to get everyone cleaned up.

My first patient there was Mrs. Kumcha. She was the wife of an active-duty soldier and she had undergone surgery there at the facility. Unfortunately, bless her heart, that surgery had gone wrong. She ended up being a quadriplegic, and it was awful. I remember that she would cluck at me. She was Korean, and she would manipulate us by making us think she didn't understand us. In truth, she really knew everything that was happening around her, if she was in the right position. She had a respirator, and we would have to turn her, of course, and reposition her every two hours. She knew, absolutely knew, when that two hours was up, and she would cluck at you to get you to come. You could not be late.

They had her in the front bed. It was an open bay area right across from the nurse's desk. We would turn her back and forth and she hated when we would turn her toward the window, because she'd end up facing away from the nurse's desk and couldn't see what was going on. Of course, then she would cluck louder. Now I know how frustrating it must have been for her, but back then, being nineteen years old, I didn't quite understand that part.

After LPN school, I ended up on a telemetry floor. That's a step down from the ICU. They didn't let new LPN graduates work there, but the ICU was where I had wanted to go. Actually, the telemetry unit turned out to be okay. I learned a lot about cardiac rhythms and about CPR. This was in the late '80s, and doctors were using a drug called quinidine to treat high blood pressure, lower the risk of heart attacks, and to slow and control the heart rhythm if a person had ventricular tachycardia. One of the side effects of that medication is elongated QR interval. When you looked at the heart rhythm on the monitor, the line looked like it was going in a circle.

Our telemetry unit had an open bay, and this one day I was sitting there with a registered nurse. We had six patients on monitors. Our boss, Staff Sergeant Easley, was in charge of us, but she wasn't there at the time. So the RN took three and I took three. When you were watching the monitors, you could raise your head and look directly at any one of your patients. Suddenly, I saw that circle rhythm start up on one of my monitors.

Now I had seen all kinds of heart rhythms, but I had never seen anything like that, and I thought the monitor was malfunctioning. But then I peered over and saw that one of my patients was blue from his neck up, and I thought, *Jeez Louise, he looks like he's having a seizure. That's not good.* The RN was relatively new as well. She hadn't been on that unit too much longer than I had, and I said, "Do you see what I see? I think we need to call a code." So she did and we started CPR. I had never seen anything like that before, so that's an early memory that sticks in my head.

From San Antonio, I went to Germany, and worked for ninety days on an inpatient drug rehab unit. Then I worked in the ER for about eighteen months and ended up in the ICU during Desert Storm, that short war in the early '90s. This may sound funny, but it was while

I was in Germany that I started questioning myself about being a nurse. I was only an LPN and, in my mind, I wasn't fully committed to spending my life as a nurse. I spent some sleepless nights, weighing my options, but after I came back from Germany, I completed my associate's degree and became a two-year RN.

However, I was still on active duty, and the Army changed its policy in the early '90s to stipulate that its RNs must hold a bachelor's of science in nursing. If I wanted to be an RN, I had to leave the service and work as a civilian or go and get my BSN. At that point, I wasn't ready to leave the Army. When I was transferred to Madigan Army Medical Center in Washington State, I didn't feel like I could prepare for the next three BSN clinicals, so I ended up switching over and getting my bachelor's of science in psychology in 2000. I wanted to continue on and earn an MSN, but the Army kept moving me – from Madigan back to San Antonio, then to Korea, and once again back to Madigan for a serious surgery. My head was spinning from all the time shifts.

After the surgery, I was fixed and deployable, as they say, but I wanted to be fit for duty near my family for a change, and they were all in Kansas. Fortunately, I was permitted to transfer to Fort Leavenworth in May 2004. This is where I finished out my military career and transitioned to my civilian job in the Family Medicine Clinic at Munson.

Sometimes now, when I get angry patients who come in because their meds didn't get refilled, or something like that, I remember Staff Sergeant Easley, my old boss on the telemetry unit. During my second stint in San Antonio, after I got promoted, I became what they call an Army Ward Master, and they moved me onto a hematology/oncology floor to be the Ward Master there. Unfortunately, Staff Sergeant Easley, who had gotten promoted to Sergeant First Class in the time since I had last seen her almost ten years earlier, was a patient on that floor. She had been diagnosed with breast cancer, and they tried a bone-marrow transplant but had failed.

The Army is very rigid in its rules sometimes. They had very strict visiting hours on the floors. But because I was the Ward Master, I was in charge, and I didn't like that rule. I didn't think it was right in that environment, where you have patients who are dying, and you're supposed to tell them, "I'm sorry. Your family member has to leave." I didn't think that was a compassionate rule. That ward was open bay also, but we had one room that was a private room, off the nurse's station, and Staff Sergeant Easley was in that room. Her family had driven from Houston to see her, and it didn't make any sense to make them leave at a specific hour. I told my staff, "Close the door, and let them stay, even if they want to stay all night with her, and leave them alone."

One day after that, I was taking care of her myself. I didn't have to work with patients on the ward, but I liked staying clinically proficient. I was doing the early-morning clean-up regimen, and I called her Sergeant Easley. She touched my hand and she said, "Just call me Margaret." But I had always called her Sergeant Easley. That's what we do in the Army. We call you by your rank. "It's okay," she said. "You can call me Margaret." That was a quiet moment, but it wasn't an ordinary one. It was very special. Sometimes you don't get a chance to connect with patients like that, or even with people in general. But Margaret had opened the door and provided that opportunity. She wanted connection. She knew she wasn't long for this earth, and she wanted to be recognized as Margaret – for the person she was.

I look back now over all the twists and turns in my career, and I'm still surprised that I chose to be a nurse. As a child, I had never dreamed of being one. As a matter of fact, I was scared to death of hospitals when I was young. A lot of people I knew went to them and never came home. I was extremely close to my grandfather, and I had a good friend for whom I babysat, and they had both died in hospitals. It's no wonder I didn't trust them. Even when I was first assigned to that female surgical floor, with Mrs. Traficante, I still hadn't overcome my fear of hospitals. But there she was, this amazing person who clearly loved what she did, and I wanted to be like her. For years, I felt afraid that I wasn't able to be a good nurse, and that I had just fallen into the job, simply because of that childhood fear of hospitals.

However, it was a patient who helped me change. When I told her about those feelings and shared my impatience with some of the junk that nurses have to do, she said, "Sometimes it's not what you want to be. It's what you're called to be." That resonated in me, and I began to understand that everyone may be called to a profession, but you have to be willing to listen for that message. You have to take it in, truly.

I have finally come to realize that nursing is my calling, and I've chosen to believe that I belong in it. I'm very blessed that I found out. It's almost like a relief. All that searching for who you're supposed to be – it's like running in quicksand. Until you really recognize who you are and what you're supposed to do and be, life can be exhausting. So now when my patients in the family clinic storm in to complain because they're angry, because they're not feeling well or, basically, because they need someone to connect with them in the simple way that Margaret connected with me, I remember, "Just call me Margaret," and that helps.

JOHN SUMMERS

I have been in the nursing profession since 1980. In my career, I have worked in a number of areas, from OB to ICU. I am presently the Director of Nursing at a sixty-eight-bed mental health facility. I have enjoyed every minute of my career, and it's difficult to pick one area that I enjoyed more than the rest.

After I got my RN license, I worked in Reno at what used to be Washoe Medical Center in its skilled nursing facility, which is the same as a nursing home. I was in charge of that for a couple of years in the early '90s. Then I went through a divorce and moved to another facility in Fallon. My title there was Director of the Alzheimer's Unit, and at the time it was the largest one in Nevada. I took that job because I was able to have a lot of patient contact, and that made it tolerable to be administration.

Many of our patients there suffered with Alzheimer's. We had one lady, and I can't say her name, but she was my welcoming committee there, and my cruise director. She had deluded herself into believing she was on an endless cruise. She would take everybody who came in, introduce the maître d' to the waitresses, show passengers to their cabins, and tell everyone what to expect on the trip. It was a pretty benign fantasy, and it was very helpful at times. She of course had Alzheimer's, and her daily reality was that cruise ship. It was actually blocking out a traumatic event, which included rape and pregnancy for her. She opted to put herself in a pleasant place and she remained there for a couple of years.

Alzheimer's is an insidious disease. We know what it is, but we're not sure what causes it. The actual diagnosis is "senile dementia of an Alzheimer's type." While you're alive, there's actually no true diagnosis that you have the condition. The only way to prove it is with an autopsy. Essentially, it results from plaque buildup in the brain, and that plaque helps to erase the memories. If you can imagine your life as a recording, like an old VHS cassette, you turn it on at birth and it starts recording. When you get near the end of your life, if Alzheimer's is at work, your tape begins to rewind. So the most recent events are soon completely gone. The longer-term memories stay with you longer. You go to bed, wake up the next day, and you don't remember your name. I took all of the mirrors off my unit because people would be scared to death when they got up in the morning and saw somebody they didn't recognize looking back at them.

At one time or another, you know, we've been told that everything is bad for us: soft drinks, Teflon pans, fatty fluids, Vitamin E, single-malt scotch, aluminum, coffee, even tap water. Now add to that list everything you can digest, including peanut butter, and you'll have what somebody somewhere once claimed as a possible cause for Alzheimer's. When I worked with senile dementia patients in the '90s, families were desperate for hope. If they had a loved one with the condition and somebody told them, "Toilet water mixed with ketchup will cure Alzheimer's," then by God – they'd try it.

We had this one old fellow who was 104 years old. He had been a private and a cook in World War I, but in his mind he had become the Supreme General – the highest-ranking military official in the world. When you're dealing with dementia or with Alzheimer's patients, there are really no therapies that have been proven effective except for validation therapy. Wherever that patient is, is fine. So if thinks he's the Supreme General, you call him that. My cruise director was the Cruise Director – that's what she was called. That's what they truly believed. You never tried to do any reality therapy with them, because they'd get very angry.

The Supreme General was absolutely adorable and, at times, even lucid. In Fallon, they have a very large naval air station, and every Memorial Day we would get their color guard to come over. We'd do a little parade around the facility, and the color guard would stop and salute the Supreme General. And he would, at 104, get up out of his wheelchair with very little assistance and snap a salute back. You could just see him light up.

Over the years, my attitude about Alzheimer's has evolved: I've gone from thinking how horrible a thing the condition is to actually believing it's not so bad for the people who have it. But it's horrible for their families. Most of the time, people who have it don't really know they have it. However, when a husband of fifty years comes into a room and his wife sitting on the bed doesn't recognize him, that can be devastating.

In 1997, my aunt was diagnosed with a terminal disease. That meant I stopped working and took care of her. In my family, that's what we did. My mother was a nurse and literally, at six years old, when I started helping her change my little brother's diapers, I knew I wanted to be one, too. She had three kids in eleven months, so she certainly needed the extra hands. I was the oldest boy, and I guess I just liked doing it. Go figure. This aunt was my mom's sister. Mom had seven kids, Aunt Sue had five, and all of us had grown up around each other. Aunt Sue had helped me through my first divorce. I used to go down and spend the weekend with her, and she'd snap me back to reality. My mother and I alternated going down and back to help her, and Aunt Sue passed in late 1997.

All through my career, I've dealt with death. I started in this business in 1980 as an orderly on an oncology med-surg floor, so death was pretty common for me there. I was initially extremely scared of it, but I found that I could handle it. Early on, I was working the night shift and one of our patients was close to death. I asked the nurse if I could sit with her until she died, because I had to know if I could deal with it. So I sat with her, holding her hand, until she took her last breath. I stayed there for several minutes afterwards, reflecting on what I had just witnessed, and I found a peace in death I hadn't known was there. I knew then that I was going to be able to handle that side of nursing.

After Aunt Sue died, I took a few months off, kind of just to relax and be reflective. Then I worked locally in Reno for a hospice company for a few years. When you meet patients who come on service in hospice, you know they have a terminal diagnosis, of course. Your job as a nurse is to make what time you have with them better time for them – whether it's taking away their pain, giving them a cold washcloth for their face, whatever it is. It's more than being of service, and it can be emotionally exhausting. So around the end of 1999, I needed a change. I still worked hospice, but I cut back my hours. By answering a crazy ad that I saw in the paper in Reno, I ended up doing what eventually got me to where I am now. That ad was, in big bold print: RNs: MAKE FIVE THOUSAND DOLLARS A WEEK. And I said, "Yeah, sure."

But I called them. I filled out an application for this company, and I didn't hear back from them for some time. Then I got a phone call one night around seven or eight o'clock in the evening, and a gentleman asked me if I would like to go to Boston and work. I said, "Really?" And he said, "Yes." And then he told me how much money I would be making.

They had a plane reservation all ready for me at nine o'clock the next morning. I called my mom and asked her to take care of my cat and my apartment. I called work and told them I was taking a week off. Then I flew to Boston and worked my first strike in Worcester, Massachusetts. That's how I became a nursing scab, and it turned out to be a little bit more than the $5,000 a week the guy had mentioned on the phone. I'll tell you what – I was happy. I worked for a week, loved it so much that I flew back home and quit my job in hospice, and then I stayed on the road for quite some time after that.

That company, U.S. Nursing, would fly nurses in from all over the country. We'd walk in and take over a hospital when they went on strike. When they figured out their problems and worked to a resolution, we'd fly out. We took over the hospital, cared for the patients, and did everything that needed to be done. Obviously, we had to be bused through picket lines and some people were a little nervous about the strikers. I wasn't ever nervous. I never felt threatened in any way, shape, or form while I was working a strike. I guess being six feet seven and weighing 350 pounds doesn't hurt, as far as that goes. I'm not your typical nurse – I don't look good in a white skirt.

Nurses on strike sounds to me like Skinemax – it's not a real scary thing – it sounds more like soft porn. And although the stories are out there about gunshots outside the hospitals and things like that, it never happened to me. I worked with some of the best nurses I've ever seen in my life. You had hundreds and hundreds of nurses coming from all over the world, with different backgrounds, different specialties, different everything. They walked into a hostile situation, and their only focus was to take care of patients. There was no gossip; there was no backstabbing; there was no whining. It was, "Let's go to work. Let's take care of the folks. Let's go home." The only thing that disgusted me was the way some of the disgruntled professionals acted when they went out on strike, destroying records and causing pain to patients.

Most of the hospitals that experience strikes have insurance, and they have to pick up the bill for everything. We made more money because we came in under hostile conditions. And for the most part, you work a lot. On a strike, you work, you go home, you go to bed, and you go back to work. The standard work week for a strike is seven twelve-hour shifts when the strike starts. Then, as the strike continues, your hours go down but your salary remains the same. It's not every week that you'll get to work, but I think in that first six months, I made somewhere in the seventy to eighty thousand dollar range.

Every time I worked a strike, every statistic was improved – in patient satisfaction and patient care. We set records for emergency room visits. And every strike that I went on, our crew was ravaged by the hospitals to pick up nurses who were better than anybody they had seen. On the Stanford strike, we lost three nurses to the heart team there. It's pretty impressive when the Stanford heart transplant team wants you to join them. Those nurses were just the hottest around.

I did strike nursing until 2004, so I was on the road roughly five years. My last job ended me up in the Bay Area and I haven't left. In between strikes, most of us would travel and take thirteen-week assignments around the country. I had a Ford F-350 four-door truck and a thirty-six-foot fifth wheel. I would take a three-month assignment somewhere and I'd park my fifth wheel near the hospital and have a grand old time. It was fun, and not bad for a single guy. I was popular for a while.

Then I decided my life needed more action, so I moved into psychiatric nursing. From 2004 until 2010, I worked at Alameda County Medical Center, in its Psychiatric Emergency Room, and that was more than an intense job. Literally, there were bloody fights almost every day. We had a doctor murdered – beaten to death by a very large female patient. The doctor was East Indian and the patient was American Indian, and the doctor ended up having a crushed trachea.

A couple of other staff got stabbed. Two of my friends were put in the hospital and had to have major reconstructive surgery. It was a war zone there: murderers, rapists, child molesters – just horrendous clientele that were picked up off the streets of Oakland and dumped on us. They were usually so high on drugs that they didn't know what they were doing when they were brought into our unit. Supposedly, they were all searched by the police before they got there, but I found many weapons and way too many drugs.

I ran the emergency room on the night shift, and every night when I got there, I went to the other in patient units to see who was working. I needed to know who was going to respond, and whether I was going to be safe that night. There were nights that I was a little frightened, but I never feared for my life. I took a couple of knives off of guys, but there was usually at least one other person on who could help. I trusted that, if we got into something bad, we could take care of whatever business we had to. I had been a cop in the Air Force before I became a nurse, and the hand-to-hand combat training I learned there was useful more than once.

If I had my guys on, then we had a group. And if that group was there, nothing happened. If one or two of us were gone, then the shit hit the fan. It took a year or a year and a half for most of the clientele to realize that, if I was working, they'd better be nice. Literally, some of the patients who were frequent fliers would tell other patients not to act up if I was in the building. They would stop them if they got too crazy. Obviously, we weren't abusive, but we were really quick to react and to stop any harmful behavior.

There was one time I was just coming into work, so it was around midnight when I walked into the ER. There was a regular named John there, taking his clothes off and making guttural sounds. Taking his clothes off was strange behavior for John, and he had six or seven people, including two police officers, surrounding him. John had initially been 5150'd, which meant he had been admitted on a three-day psychiatric hold, for running around on BART in underroos, claiming to be Spiderman. John thought he was a superhero and he was always in fights, on the streets and in the facility. In the psychiatric world, patients have the right to wear their own clothing, so John was allowed to keep his Spiderman outfit.

After our first couple of meetings, John had started calling me The Incredible Hulk. So The Hulk and Spiderman became fast friends. No matter how high he was, and no matter what situation he was in – and there were a couple – he would stop everything and give me a hug. Well, that particular night, everyone was just ready to fight, and I walked in and started laughing my head off. I said, "Johnny, come here. Put your damned clothes on." And he did. The looks on the faces of the staff were priceless. They just couldn't believe it. I told them, "Superheroes, you know? We have to stick together."

John and I never really fought, but there were several guys who came in and all they wanted to do was fight. They'd attack. They'd swing and kick and bite and scratch and spit, and what happened was they were put down hard and fast. If you attacked one of my staff when I was on duty, you went into restraints, and you were given a very large dose of medication that basically knocked you unconscious.

The worst fight I was in probably involved me, two police officers, and a client. This client, who had a history of felony assaults, was a nasty, aggressive man, and completely psychotic. He had been in and out of jail most of his forty years. The police officers were stationed there because he was under arrest. In the bathroom, though, he made a jailhouse club – which is a sock with whatever heavy object that you can put in it – and he came out swinging. He had some change in there and some soap and a couple of full, little mouthwash bottles. They were enough to give it good weight, and it took all three of us to subdue him. It wasn't until the floor and the walls were bloody and two of us were hurt – one of the police officers and me – that we got him under control. We weren't badly hurt, but still, that's a lot of fight for one guy. He was big, but the cops were healthy fellows, too. But this guy just came out swinging that club. We defended ourselves, and we jumped him. The cops had their batons out, and we dropped him on the floor, choking him out. They kicked him in the ribs and hit him with the batons, but he just wouldn't quit. He was really psychotic.

When we were done with him, of course I immediately started tending to his wounds, and he thanked me for the ass-whipping. He actually said, "I probably needed that. I appreciate it." And off he went to the hospital. That's just how bizarre it was. There was almost no time for nursing because you had to defend yourself all the time. That's the biggest reason that I eventually left. I was tired of not being able to nurse people.

I actually got head-hunted for my current job. I'm the Director of Nurses for Telecare Cordilleras. It's a sixty-eight-bed mental health recovery center. We also have a forty-nine-bed residential program as well, in the same building. Telecare Company is really big in the Bay Area and on the West Coast for psychiatric nursing. It's a little bit new to me, but what I've tried to do in the last year is change the whole culture of the facility because, before I got here, there had not been a director of nursing for over seven months. I've got by far the largest department in this facility. I've got over sixty staff, and that staff, without leadership, and as people normally do, rose to their level of incompetence. And there were some very high levels here.

My first ten months were spent putting out brush fires and trying to fix things that were broken. Every once in a while, we have a glitch in one of the systems that I've put in, but for the most part, there's not a lot that's broken anymore. Now we're just working on fine-tuning some of the attitudes and re-energizing people to get back to why they wanted to be nurses in the first place. Psychiatric nursing is a very difficult job for people to stay energized in. It's tough dealing with the mentally challenged. We still have assaults here. We still have people who yell and scream 24/7, and when you have sixty-eight clients who are all doing that, it can drain you. We're a recovery-based program, so we're working toward getting people to a lower level of care.

Since I've been here, we've discharged clients who have been here for fifteen to twenty years to lower levels of care. We still have one who has been here for 4200 days, and another who has been here over 3000 days. But we're working hard to reduce the number of long-term, chronic patients so we can handle more short-term, six-months-a-year kinds of clients.

I've known all my life that, without nurses, you don't have a hospital. Unfortunately, nurses take the brunt of everybody's anger: if the system's wrong, it's the nurse's' fault. That's kind of what had been happening here. Well, nurses are a very nutty group of people. If you're a nurse, and somebody who isn't a nurse tells you what to do, we will chew you up and spit you out. So they had non-nursing personnel trying to direct nurses. We don't get directed well by non-nurses. It's a little bit of a respect thing, but it's a fact also that, by law, you can't tell me what to do. If I do what you say in regard to patient care, and it's wrong, then it's my license and I can go to jail.

When I got here, these nurses had no direction; they had no leadership. So it's taken me the better part of the last year to move that kind of thinking – *Oh, it's the nurses' fault* – to *How can we help the nurses?* And I'm making sure that I communicate to my nurses that, "Guess what, guys? You're it. You're the ones who decide things. You get to do things the way that nurses are supposed to do them." I'm doing things here that most directors of nursing don't get to do, and that's making this department mine. It will take on my personality.

I love to teach, and I've been able to teach everybody here a lot of things, because I've got as much of a medical background as I do a psychiatric background. So I've been able to use a lot of those skills. It's just fun now being able to actually direct the path of the nursing department. For thirty years, I've been directed, and now I'm directing that path. This facility and this company are doing some really cutting-edge stuff with psychiatric nursing, and it's a real treat to be on the ground floor and trying to build something good.

After thirty-two years of nursing, I still love doing it. During all that time, I have never once NOT wanted to go to work. And I may only know you as a patient for three days, but in those three days, I may change your life. Certainly in those three days, if I've got you on a med-surg floor or something like that, I will make your life better. Knowing that I can be of that kind of service to people is what makes nursing as much fun as it is for me.

Here's what I mean. Back in 1982 at St. Mary's, early in my career, I met a big old country boy, Larry. He didn't have any teeth, he did have a mullet, and he was a forty-something-year-old truck driver. Larry also had leukemia. One of the best technical nurses that I've ever seen in my life was the nurse that I was working with that night, and he went in to explain to Larry his newly diagnosed leukemia. Back then, that was a death sentence.

Well, Larry wasn't what he would call an "edumacated fella." He had no clue what this nurse had told him, because the nurse had gotten very technical. I walked in after that and saw the dumbfounded look on his face. He said, "Pardon my French." – and I quote – "What the fuck did he just say?" I looked at him and laughed and said, "Larry, you've got cancer in your blood, and you're going to die." And he said, "Well, why in the hell didn't he say that?"

For the next two months, every night that I worked and he was able, Larry and I would sit in his room and we would talk about women and drinking and truck driving and old country-boy stuff. We didn't talk about death or dying or nursing or anything else. Every once in a while, I'd bring him a beer, and we'd sit and drink a beer together. That was okay with the doctors. And Larry, just shortly before he died, shook my hand and said, "Thank you. You've made me better." Then he died. He was not there the next night when I came to work.

That was a career-maker: one of those moments with a patient when the connection is so intense, and on such a visceral level, that neither of you will ever forget it. I certainly never did. You can't do a better job than that as a nurse, and I can't imagine myself doing anything more worthwhile.

MELISSA ERICKSON

I worked in Women Care at a large hospital in Minneapolis which delivers more babies than any other hospital in the state. Women Care is a level IV obstetric care facility. Primarily I cared for high-risk mothers and babies there, including high-order multiples. In May 2010, I took a new position of OB Educator and since then I have obtained my BSN, PHN, and MSN Ed. degrees.

My mom had multiple sclerosis. She was diagnosed right after I was born, when she was about twenty-two. The diagnosis for MS back then was very hard to differentiate, and she had probably been sick with it prior to that for many years. As a child, I saw her have horrible symptoms. She would have paralysis. One day, all of a sudden, her hand would just develop contracture and she would become paralyzed on one side. Or I remember once, when I was five, she became blind. That lasted for about a month. MS is neurological. It can do anything to a person. The full gamut of anything that could go wrong did.

I think her condition made me resist wanting to be a nurse. I thought, *Maybe I shouldn't do this because it's too hard to care for somebody.* My perception of caring for sick and needy people was a little bit different because of those painful experiences with my mom. When you live with it, it's often harder than it is at a job, where you can go to work, deal with problems for eight hours, and then go home. A lot of depression and emotional issues accompany caregiving with your family. But also, when you grow up around somebody with a chronic disability, becoming a caregiver is how you survive, so that becomes a part of who you are, too.

When I was about twelve, I experienced a traumatic event with my mother. We were camping in northern Wisconsin. She was standing on the top step of our camper, and then she lost her balance. Vertigo was one of the primary symptoms of her MS, and she lost her balance frequently. She fell backwards and landed on her head only a few feet from where I stood, and lay there unconscious and unresponsive. All I could do was scream. I didn't know what else to do, and the fact that I didn't know what to do, or how to help her, became the most traumatic part of the experience for me.

I felt relatively helpless around my mom's disease until I was in ninth grade, and then things started to change. The high school I attended offered a program called OEC, Opportunities in Emergency Care, and through that program I obtained my EMT license when I was fifteen. After I got my license, I chose the postsecondary enrollment option, which is where you go to college instead of high school, and I took all my prerequisites for the nursing program. I did it half time for my junior year and full time for my senior year. So when I graduated from high school, I basically had my associate in science degree. That was great. Two years of college basically for free is a good thing.

Then I tried different things for a while to see what I wanted to do. I felt like I had to be sure. I tried everything. I even became an insurance agent. And then I finally decided to enroll in a private college. *Teaching would be a good career*, I thought. *That's still caring for people.* I had been running classes in first aid and EMS at the time and I enjoyed interacting with students. So I was studying to be a teacher when – the typical story – I met a guy, we decided to get married, and I had a baby.

During college and the early years of my marriage, I fell back on my EMT license, providing emergency medical services for employees at the *Minneapolis Star Tribune* newspaper. I worked the night shift, and my husband worked at his job during the day. There was always around-the-clock emergency care for all the staff and, at night, when all the presses ran, often I would be the only female in the building. There would be from 100 to 300 men in there, and I'd provide occupational health care and emergency support if they needed anything. They called me the nurse, and that role started to stick.

The *Star Tribune* would hire homeless people from the streets on Saturday nights. They were the ones who folded the advertisements into the Sunday paper. So Saturday night was always an interesting one at work because not only did you have regular staff there, but you also had all the homeless people with their many needs. For their breaks, where did they go? They went to the nurse's office, usually, or they tried to find a warm place to sleep. Sometimes it was just that they needed to talk to someone.

It was during that time I made my mind up about nursing. Being an EMT didn't pay very well and I decided that if I had to work and be away from my kids, I needed to make it worth my while. So I enrolled in a distance education program. The only requirement that I had to take, in addition to the core nursing program, was microbiology. The *Star Tribune* actually supported me and paid for some of my education with excellent tuition reimbursement.

I worked nights, I went to school, and I had kids. That was my life. I didn't sleep much back then. I would get home usually around 4:00 a.m. and sleep until the kids got up, usually around 7:00, and that was it. Three hours a night, average, for many years. All the hard work paid off, though: I graduated in 1998, when I was twenty-five, and I got licensed in Minnesota as an RN soon after.

I stayed at the *Star Tribune* for – let me see, I think about this in babies – I was on my third baby at that point. So it must have been five or six years. Then I took an RN job at a county hospital out in the country. We moved quite a ways west of Minneapolis then, and in that hospital I was required to work in all areas of the hospital and in the ER. That's when I started doing OB care. I never thought for a minute that would be where I'd end up. I always thought it was going to be the ER because of my EMT experience. I fell into the OB thing and it just evolved into a kind of calling. You know I think it might have been because, when I had my first baby, I was so completely terrified. I didn't have anyone who really helped me through that, and I thought, *Well, I could help moms have their babies and make that process easier for them.* And the feedback I got from my patients was that I did help them. I'd get that hug afterwards, or they'd ask me to stay late after my shift, just to be with them. When that happens, it's obvious you're having a positive influence.

I remember my first week in the OB unit there I had a patient who was having her fifteenth baby. She was probably in the thirty-eight to forty-two range, so that would have meant she had a baby about every fifteen months or something. There are two religious groups out there, both of them Lutheran, that do not believe in using any form of birth control. That woman had a daughter who was across the hall in another delivery room, having her own baby, and they were both about to deliver at the same exact time – and this was in a tiny rural hospital. I was trying to run back and forth to monitor both patients, and family members were all over the place, and I remember feeling kind of floored and wondering, *What do I do next?* So that was my introduction.

I grew up in the city, and I was used to ER-type work. It was really hard for me to stay out there in the country. There were moments of real activity, but often I longed for a faster pace. So I took a job with Women Care at a large hospital in Minneapolis. They handled more births than any other hospital in the state. Women Care was a Level IV obstetric care facility – that's the highest level OB care possible. From Minnesota, Wisconsin, the Dakotas, and Iowa, all the difficult cases were flown into us at that facility. We took care of quads, triplets, and even sextuplets. High-order multiples, unusual pregnancies – anything that normal places wouldn't treat, we dealt with there.

Perinatologists are specialists in high-risk, maternal-fetal medicine and, at that hospital, we had the largest group of them in the country. That's why we attracted so many complicated cases. Here's an alarming fact that underscores the sometimes hopeless, high-risk cases that were sent to us: there were so many deaths on our OB unit that they had to provide a chaplain specifically for our staff and patients.

Women Care was on the hospital's top two floors, on the fifth and sixth floors, and there were about 160 RNs working there. I think there were about forty or forty-five postpartum rooms, and sixteen labor rooms. We also had a high-risk ante-partum unit, which was where we would put patients who were either more stable or long-term, because a lot of women would stay with us for months before they delivered. And so they would be down on that unit, which could hold about fourteen patients.

When I started there, it was not uncommon to be assigned the whole wing of the postpartum unit, and that meant couplet care – moms and babies. So we would have to care for up to eight moms and babies – that meant at least sixteen RN head-to-toe assessments – and you had to chart on each one, along with doing all the nighttime stuff and feeding and bringing babies in and out of the nursery constantly. It was chaos.

But the nurses there were the best nurses I've ever worked with. You never had a shortage of help whenever you needed it. I'd put on the call light and say, "I need help in here," and I'd have five people running right in. I was still the one responsible for doing the charting and all that, but I had tons of help whenever a situation was happening.

I was there when one of our high-order multiples was delivered prematurely, and that situation was wrong from the start. We're talking about very tiny babies. The mom was posting pictures on the Internet of her getting up, walking around, doing all this stuff, when she was supposed to be on bed rest. She was posting about how much money she would make when she signed an agreement with the news media. There we were, struggling to do everything we could to help her, and she should have been doing everything she could to maintain the health of her babies. That is not the kind of thing you want people doing. It seemed planned and purposeful. We all told her that there was a much greater chance of mortality the quicker she delivered.

I was blunt with her. I said, "Here's the deal. If you don't do what we're telling you, you're going to have these babies way too early. They're either going to be born and be underdeveloped and have multiple medical problems, or they're going to die. Your odds of your babies surviving at twenty-two weeks is about 20 percent. That's not including the problems with cerebral palsy and all the other things that can go along with that." She didn't listen.

She delivered at twenty-two weeks and five days, and her babies were micro-preemies – less than a pound. Out of the babies who were born, only one survived, and he was on a ventilator. If she wanted to sell her story to the news media and win her pot of gold and fifteen minutes of fame, what she found out was that nobody will buy a story where you have multiple funerals.

I could tell you hundreds of birth stories: a mother who had amniotic band syndrome, where part of the amnion leaked and wrapped around her baby's feet and hands, or another mom with aplastic anemia who went into a coma while pregnant, when her baby demised in utero. Although we performed a C-section to save her life, she didn't survive either. There are many, many others, but it becomes overwhelming to talk about them.

No matter what happened, though, most women wanted to have pictures of their lost babies as part of their mourning process. We worked with an organization called Now I Lay Me Down to Sleep, which had been started by a woman who was a professional photographer and whose own baby had died. Now that kind of job takes a really special person. Those photographers who came in were awesome. All of them had suffered a loss of their own, so they could relate to the grieving mothers. They were super sensitive to them.

Very rarely did I bring the job home with me, but it was so intense that there wasn't room for much else when I did get home. I was just exhausted from it, and occasionally I couldn't even sleep. My only coping strategy was to detach myself to a certain extent. I think I probably learned that in the EMT world because we were drilled, every single day, to put whatever we experienced aside and do our jobs – no matter what the sight or the smell or the sound.

More importantly, I have seen hundreds of healthy births, thank goodness. I have also seen many babies survive when they shouldn't have survived, and I considered them miracles. Thirty years ago, we didn't resuscitate babies if they were under thirty-two weeks. Now we do it at twenty-three weeks. So we're getting better at it. I know the smallest birth I participated in was a boy who weighed fourteen ounces. He came out crying, was put on a ventilator for about twenty-four hours, and then he was extubated. He breathed on his own and did fine.

However, enough chaos was finally enough. Now I work as an OB educator. I work with a group of general practice OB/GYNs, so it's not high-risk anymore. It's almost all normal risk. Patients find out they're pregnant, and they call the clinic for an appointment. Instead of seeing the doctor, they see me. I spend an hour with them, talking about pregnancy, about routine prenatal care, and explaining to them what they should do to have a safe and healthy baby. I hook them up with social workers if they need that. If it's an early pregnancy, the mom usually asks about nausea and vomiting. So we talk about those concerns, what you do for them, and which medications are safe in pregnancy. We talk about food safety because that's a big thing. When you're pregnant you can't eat lunch meat and you can't eat sushi or things like that because of listeriosis – the bacteria that gives you what they sometimes call stomach flu.

I usually get them an ultrasound on that first day, and do their laboratory tests. I talk to them about nutrition. If your body mass index is over 30, you're at very high risk for diabetes – that's my standard. Any of my pregnant patients who have a BMI over 30 have to take a glucose test that same day, and most of them don't pass. Probably 50 percent of the patients I see have needed an early glucose test, and almost half of them are actually diabetic. So then they begin with insulin. It's NOT gestational – not because of the pregnancy – it's just that they're truly diabetic.

What happens is, when you're diabetic and you're pregnant, your blood sugar is high and your pancreas isn't pumping out enough insulin. Your baby tries to compensate, and tries to cover the maternally-induced high blood sugar that affects it. That's how you get those ten and twelve-pound babies. Then, once the baby is born, it's used to putting out all that insulin, but now it's not getting all those calories and all the glucose. It continues to put out that insulin if it has low blood sugar, and that can be very serious. The baby can end up on an IV. So it is a big deal. They've had to increase the hours of the registered dietician and another RN diabetes educator since I started because of the tests I've been doing, but we're seeing healthier pregnancies.

I can also offer genetic testing to my patients. Out here where I am, though, it's a conservative culture. Maybe 1-2 percent of our population wants it. People usually do genetic testing for a couple of reasons: they're either a Type A personality, or they're worried that something may be wrong with the fetus. And based on that genetic information, they could consider abortion. But if they're pro-life and conservative and don't believe in birth control, they don't choose that testing.

One nice surprise in this new job is that the clinic doctors know I've worked with the best perinatologists in the region, and they do rely on my high-risk labor and delivery experience. They'll come to me and ask, "Well, what about this doctor? What does he do normally?" There have been a few high-risk situations that have occurred, and I've helped them coordinate care for those patients.

I love it when I see positive outcomes happen for my patients – when I see them making lifestyle changes that improve their health and that of their babies. And when they say, "Oh, you helped me so much the last time," it reminds me why I'm here and reassures me that what I'm doing is helping. It's that kind of reaffirmation that keeps me going.

Now is this current job something I want to do for the rest of my life? No way. It's not mentally challenging enough. But I have some more autonomy working as an educator and some extra time. Because of that extra time, I went back to school and I actually just graduated with my master's in nursing and education. Right now I'm being recruited by a couple of colleges. They want me to go and teach nursing. Most nurses are not trained in OB, so I would teach that at least, as well as anything related to reproduction or obstetrics. I love to teach, so I'll try it. And if that's not stimulating enough, I'll go back to working in a hospital.

I think nursing is a fabulous career. I believe nurses are trusted and respected more than doctors, even, but if you're going to go into this profession, you have to really care about people. Patients are putting their lives in your hands. You have to hold that responsibility close to your heart and really consider what's happening right now, every moment, every day. You have to resolve to do your absolute best for every single patient, no matter what.

CHRISTI SIEDLICKI

As a new LPN, I worked on a neurological rehab unit and then in a pediatric and neonatal ICU. I also worked for the local health department, providing family-planning counseling when it was very controversial in my area. As an RN, I worked in a clinic setting, and started my own First Call business, in which I offered pediatric telephone assessment and advice. I also played a large part in starting a tri-county sexual assault nurse examiner program that has continued to grow in the Midwest.

I was living in Grants Pass, Oregon, in the mid-'90s, working as a pediatric nurse and volunteering with the health department in Josephine County, where I offered family planning counseling. In our very conservative area, that was controversial back then. It wasn't exactly a pro-choice area. I was about twenty-two then, and a Portland reporter came down to do an article about it, and my picture ended up in the paper.

In 1998, I married a doctor who was working in Wisconsin. When I moved there, I met a nurse who had just moved there as well, and she had the bright idea to start a local sexual assault nurse examiner program. They're wonderful programs, and they're all over the country. The examiners are called SANE nurses – sexual assault nurse examiners – and they're nurses who have special training to collect forensic evidence. They collect it more gently than most ER docs, who are usually in a hurry and, honestly, are usually men. Most SANE nurses go into that field because they're following their hearts, and they want to perform the exams in a caring yet professional manner.

I took a special course and became certified. That was step one. In the meantime, my friend, Jacqui, was trying to get the program up and running. She was meeting with the district attorney and saying that we had this program ready. In reality, at that point it was just her and me, and I had only recently finished my training. But she really got me on board. I'm much more of a nuts-and-bolts-person, so I wrote our policies and procedures, and I secured a grant that provided work space. Then the "pink ladies" at one of the hospitals got us a brand new colposcope, which is a special magnifying device. After the grant and the donation, I was able to write a training program and begin hiring other nurses who would undergo the training. It actually turned into a very successful, three-county-area program in Wisconsin and Illinois that is still running today.

I did exams on kids as young as about two, and I examined women up to about forty-five or fifty. The part I liked best was that I was one of the good guys. But there was a downside, too: since I specialized in kids, I learned far too much about how many people you can't trust. Up to that point, I had been a very trusting person, and it was disillusioning for me to find out there are so many people out there who like to hurt children. That was extremely difficult.

The way it worked, I would either get the call from the police department or from the ER, depending on where the point of contact was. If the police department got the call, they would tell me that they had someone who needed an exam, and I would make the arrangements to see them right away. Oftentimes, with children, they haven't been recently assaulted. They've been molested over time, so it's not always necessary to do the exam immediately to collect evidence. With some of those kids, I could make appointments to visit them in their homes. Mostly, I would just do some playtime with them so they could get to know me and feel more comfortable. Sometimes I would meet with kids several times before I would even ask them a question. The kinds of exams that I was doing were very personal, of course, and most of the children were understandably apprehensive, so it took a while before they trusted me.

One of the times I remember best was a little girl who was about eight years old. She was school shopping with her parents one day, and she left her clothes in the car when the family went up to eat dinner. When she remembered that she had left them there, she ran down to the car to get them, and a man grabbed her. He started running off with her to a nearby field. The parents noticed she was missing almost immediately and called the police. Her dad ran out to look for her, and he was the first person to find the man who was assaulting his daughter. He gave him what for, and the police let him keep at it there for a few seconds, but he didn't kill him.

The little girl and her parents came to see me afterwards, and that was one of those instances where I had to collect the forensic evidence immediately. Now the abuser had been caught, and the little girl was safe, but she had gotten assaulted. So even though the father had literally grabbed him in the act, I still had to collect evidence. The family was remarkably calm. Even the little girl was calm. She was amazing. It was just one of those stunning moments I'll never forget.

If I had to examine an adult, I had a room where we would talk, and I would do an interview first to find out what had happened. Then I would conduct a head-to-toe exam, taking pictures and documenting everything I discovered. Oftentimes, more details of the story would be revealed or confirmed during the exam anyway. You could see the evidence on their bodies, and you could start to see fingerprints or bruises starting to appear. My first question would usually be something general, like "Tell me about what happened," and I would observe their expressions and body language. I'd be looking for clues about what to ask next. And then I had another set of questions I would ask to confirm specific times and body parts, things like that, and we would work our way down through the layers of the story.

Most of the people I examined were traumatized, as you'd expect, but most of the time they also really wanted justice. You know how when something horrifying happens to you, you go into shock and think, *Oh, my gosh, what happened*? So maybe they couldn't talk about it at first, but the longer I spent with them, the easier it became. Most of them wanted the person caught and, by consenting to the exam, they were really hoping that might ensure the person could be convicted.

We always did prophylaxis for sexually transmitted diseases, giving them antibiotics that would protect them from getting certain STDs. So we did tests for those. We also provided the morning-after pill for women who wanted to take it as a precaution against getting pregnant. Of course, that's a little controversial, too. I believe it's about giving women a choice. I can't imagine that there would be many people who were assaulted who would want to have that child. I never came across anyone who refused the pill, but I'm sure that it happens – just not in my experience.

One of the things I noticed was the way different groups reacted to the crimes. Sometimes I would be doing an exam in Madison or Milwaukee or someplace urban, and there were distinct cultural differences. For instance, women who were with Hispanic men seemed to struggle with their decisions much more because their men frequently blamed them. They acted as if the women had brought the assault on themselves, and that they were somehow tarnished by the victimization. Most of the Hispanic women I treated were very nervous about how their partners would react.

I was involved in testifying for some really important convictions. I had one very memorable case where a woman came in who had clearly been attacked. She said, "I'm just doing this because he's going to kill me, and I want everybody to know what he did before he kills me." I put her in a safe house and tried to keep her location a secret, but her husband did end up killing her. Her son told his dad where she was. That was really tragic. The rape charge was dropped as part of the plea bargain in that case so, sadly, she never got her wish. He was convicted of murder, though.

One of the things that I noticed, particularly when I was in court testifying, was that many people still wanted to believe that women were somehow responsible for instigating the violent attacks against them. It was almost like, if they could find a reason that she deserved it, and they know they wouldn't act that way, then they could remain safe. Does that make any sense? All kinds of people seemed to believe that. We would have these jury trials and, with the evidence, I would be sure that it would be a slam dunk, but that wasn't always the case.

If the defense attorney took the position that the victim had asked for it, many people really seemed to buy into that. *Look at the way she dressed. It was because she was out late at night.* The truth is that people don't ever deserve that. Women rarely ask for sexual violence against themselves. We had an incredible district attorney that we worked with, and he built strong cases. I would always be surprised when one didn't result in a conviction, and it almost always seemed like it happened when the defense took a "she-deserved-it" position.

That need to blame the victim scared me. But think about it: think about how, when you hear that somebody has died in a car accident, you ask, "Well, were they drinking? Were they wearing a seat belt? What were they doing that caused them to die in that car accident?" Because you're looking for a way that you can be safe, right? I think maybe it's the same kind of thing, but I still never agreed with it.

I worked with that sexual assault program until 2002, when I moved back to Oregon, where I was able to step right back into pediatric nursing, though in a different office. I love kids. I feel like I can relate to them. When I was in nursing school for the first go-round, thirty years ago, I loved the pediatric rotation. At the time, I thought, *You know, I'm going to come back to this.* I also like working with the parents, and I enjoy being able to reassure them that they're doing a good job. I really like the way that kids get well so fast. If you do an intervention on them to try and help them get better, you usually know right away whether it's going to work or not.

I was thinking recently, *What is it that I have learned from being a nurse that makes me well suited for the job that I do now?* I decided it's really just looking at the big picture, looking two steps ahead, noticing when there's a problem, being detail-oriented while still staying aware of the big picture – keeping my eye on all of it. When you notice that something isn't right, you have to start turning your wheels to figure it out: *How could this be better?* And then you try to fix it. It's like assembling the pieces of a puzzle.

GERALD HALLMAN

I have been involved with health care for over thirty-six years. I started as a basic EMT in 1976, and then worked as a paramedic, both on an ambulance and in a hospital, for ten years. Since I became an RN in 1991, I have been the nurse manager of a PACU in southern Georgia, a Red Cross nurse at Ground Zero, a travel nurse, an administrative supervisor for a 200-plus-bed hospital, a hospice nurse, and a director at a state facility for mentally and physically dysfunctional patients. Besides my nursing degree, I also have degrees in electronic and electromechanical engineering technology and in paralegal studies.

I didn't start out to be a nurse. In 1975, when I was twenty-three, I was working as an estimator and a draftsman at a glass company in Athens, Georgia. I went home for lunch, and when I was headed back to work on my motorcycle, an old lady made a U-turn and hit me. The bumper of her car crushed my left leg. What I didn't realize was that my tib-fib had broken just above the ankle. So, as the bike started to fall, I put that foot down to kick it back up and try to ride it out. When I did that, my foot snapped off and landed about eighteen inches away from me. I tried to get up, looked down, and thought, *Oh, crap*. I went into a state of shock, of course, but I didn't pass out. I was conscious the entire time.

A guy hurried out of a store across from where I was lying and said, "I'm going to put a tourniquet on your leg," and I told him, "No, you're not." I had been a senior scout instructor in Boy Scouts for our area, teaching first aid, since 1966. I knew that sometimes when you put a tourniquet on, everything below the tourniquet can be lost. So I showed him how to apply direct pressure on specific points and elevate the leg until the ambulance arrived.

My boss happened to be on the other side of the street. He ran over to see how I was doing, and I counted off the jobs for which I had contracts ready to be turned in, what bids were due, and what shop drawings needed to be done. He stared down at me like I was crazy, and he was right. That's just who I am.

When the EMTs finally came, I had already done my own assessment. I told them where I was injured and how badly. They put my foot and my leg together and fastened an air splint to hold them in place. The air splint put pressure all the way along the leg and controlled the bleeding without cutting it off. The way my foot was torn off twisted the blood vessels, and they basically shut themselves off, except for the major ones. Then when they put the air splint on, that actually slowed everything down enough so I was still getting some blood flow in my leg. It didn't provide any flow to my detached foot, of course, but when they put the foot inside the air splint, that kept it from losing what blood was in it. And after they packaged me up, they packed some ice around my foot to preserve it.

St. Mary's Hospital, a fairly big hospital in Athens, was only about half a mile away from where I was hit. The ER doc who first saw me said, "Son, you're going to lose your foot." I told him I wanted a second opinion. Well, there was a doctor who just happened to be walking through the hospital. His name was Hugh Hastings. He was an orthopedic surgeon, but he wasn't on duty there. He had come to the hospital to visit a friend. Somebody saw him wandering through and asked him to have a look. He picked up my foot and leg and stared hard at them. I said, "Can you put it back together?"

"Oh, yeah, I can fix it," he said.

"How are you going to do it?"

"I'll show you."

He walked out of the room, and I was expecting him to come back with bolts and screws and plates. But he walked back in with a bottle of Elmer's glue and said, "The best damned stuff that orthopedic surgeons ever invented." So I figured the guy was a nut case and I could trust my life to him. He had just as sick a sense of humor as I had. He said, "I saw worse than this in Vietnam." Turned out he had done three tours of duty in Vietnam as a M.A.S.H. doctor.

So I had my surgery and spent three days in the ICU. Between then and 1987, I had seventeen more surgeries. They took a muscle out of my back to rebuild my ankle, and I've had seven different skin grafts. But here's the important part: the EMTs who had picked me up visited me after that first surgery. "Here, sign this," they said. "It's an application to become an EMT." I started EMT school in 1975, on crutches. I graduated the next year from there, and right after that, I applied to nursing school.

Nursing was different back in 1976. Along with four other guys, I entered a regular nursing program, but all of our teachers were women, and they did not like the idea of male nurses. As a matter of fact, they told us, "There's no place in nursing for men," and none of us finished that program. They said we were incapable of caring for patients because we didn't understand how to have sympathy. There wasn't a male who graduated from that program until 1988.

So I went back and trained to be a paramedic and I got a lot of great experience working at that. At one point, St. Mary's had a nursing shortage, so they had paramedics working in their ICU. Under state law at that time, anything that was deemed emergency or critical care could be handled by a paramedic. I regularly did things on my job that RNs weren't allowed to do. If there was a code, I would intubate the patient. I could even put in chest tubes and central lines. But I still wanted to be a nurse.

One of the hospital administrators asked me if I had ever heard of the Regents program and explained that it was a way I could stay at my job but also earn my degree and become an RN. He said, "Would you be interested if we paid all the costs?" And I said, "Oh, yeah." I signed up and took my first test in May of 1990. I took all the classes and passed them, finished all my course work in 1991, and only had to pass my clinical exam. The clinical was a three-day clinical competency assessment, starting on a Friday night at Grady Hospital, which is a teaching facility. They had a nursing preceptor who would monitor you and make sure you didn't kill any patients.

So first thing on that Friday night, we did a lab, and I did fine. On Saturday, I had two different patients. One was a pediatric patient, who was dehydrated. They couldn't get him to drink anything. I walked in and spent about ten minutes just talking to him. Then I went down to the cafeteria and came back with a bath pan full of juices, all on ice. He took and drank all of them. He told me he didn't like water, didn't like milk, but he loved juice. By the end of the day, he was rehydrated. The preceptor said to me, "How'd you know to do that?" And I said, "I've got kids. I'm a dad."

On Sunday, I was supposed to have my last patient. I got there at 6:00 a.m. to review all the information. I was sitting there, reading the EKG, and my preceptor was watching me. The doctor for that patient came in and said, "Do you have his EKG?" I said, "Yeah, but I want to show you something," and I pointed out the rhythm. I said, "Look, you prescribed this medication. It's okay, but it would be better if you changed it." I explained how the rhythm would improve if it were treated with a different medication, and he said, "Okay, you're right." He took the chart, rewrote his orders and, after that, the rest of my exam went off without a hitch. All I had to do then was take the state boards and, as soon as I got my license, I was hired as a charge nurse at the hospital where I had been working as a paramedic.

We had twenty-eight beds on that neuro-surgical unit, and four or five nurses working. I had been there maybe six to eight months when one of the nurses who had given me the most grief when I was in that first nursing program came walking down the hall. She said, "Oh, I guess you're one of the orderlies here. I need to speak to the charge nurse." And I said, "You are."

"What do you mean?" she said.

"I am the charge nurse. What do you want?"

"Well, I want to put my nurses down here so they can learn what to do about neuro-surgical."

And I told her, "That's fine. Your students can come, but you can't. I don't trust your judgment. I think it's flawed."

"Well, I'll speak to your manager."

My manager came out and listened to her complaints. My manager just looked at her and said, "If Gerald says he doesn't trust you, that's good enough for me. Your students can come, but you can't."

Oh, that was sweet.

After that, they wanted me to transfer down to the recovery room – to the post-anesthesia care unit. We saw a variety of critical-care patients in that PACU. We saw patients who had undergone open-heart surgery or severe kinds of trauma, and we took care of them the way we would in an ICU. But after we finished with them, we sent them along to somebody else.

My first day on the job in the PACU, I put in eighteen hours. My boss was sitting there, and she said, "You're not coming back, are you?" And

I said, "Oh, yeah, I like this. This is fun." She stared at me and said, "You think this is fun?" What was fun for me about it was the adrenaline rush. It's the same thing as when you're a paramedic and you get that call – trauma, wreck, gunshot, whatever. The old adrenaline gets cranking, and you're thinking at faster-than-light-speed, and it really pumps you up. Everything becomes crystal clear and you can make snap decisions, and that's a lot of fun. You have to really keep up with the pumps, the drips, and everything else to keep someone alive.

We had a patient once who was a literal train wreck: he was in a vehicle that had gotten hit by a train. We got him on a Friday night just around midnight. He had already been in surgery for about ten hours before they brought him to us in the PACU. He had bilateral chest contusions. We had rotating chest tubes, where we'd clamp it for fifteen minutes and then release it for fifteen minutes – on both sides. We couldn't let it keep draining; we had to relieve the pressure. We were hanging all kinds of fluids and blood because he kept bleeding out. His ribs had punctured his lungs, and they had to piece him back together during the surgery.

We had an anesthesiologist, a CRNA, a pulmonologist, and a cardiac surgeon, along with me and another nurse, all standing at this guy's bedside the whole time. The docs would take catnaps on a stretcher next to him. We did that from about 2:00 a.m. on Saturday until 6:00 p.m. on Sunday. Believe it or not, he survived.

We had another patient, an eighteen-year-old kid who had gone face first through a plate glass window. He was sliced from the front of his neck almost all the way back to his spine. He cut his right carotid and his right internal and external jugular, and he lost 80 percent of his blood on the scene. When they brought him to the OR, as they were doing compressions on him, his blood was a light pink color. It was more IV fluids than blood.

As a PACU nurse, I would often go back and help them get a case started, and then I would get things ready for when the patient came into recovery. In that particular case, I held the patient's jugulars and carotid together with my hands and let the doctor stitch them to stabilize him. After that, I helped the ET team keep his lungs going.

Now at the same time, we had a guy who had been transferred from a smaller hospital near Athens. He had just been in the wrong place at the wrong time, and someone had cut him across his abdomen so deep that his intestines had spilled out. They were packed in a plastic bag, lying on top of his stomach, when he reached us. So we had to stuff those back in and sew him up. For a while, it was really nuts in there with those two severe traumas.

Well, the next day, that kid who had gone through the window actually opened his eyes, responded to questions, followed commands, squeezed our hands, and recognized his parents when they finally got there. Before I left to go home, I took his parents aside and said, "Look, I don't care what your religious beliefs are. It's none of my business. But I need to tell you one thing. You need to get your checkbook and find your minister and write a check for any tithing you have not yet paid. You owe God; you do not owe us. We didn't think he'd make it out of the OR. Stamp an "M" on that boy and call him "miracle." And after he recovered, he had less than a 5 percent loss of function. That's all. It was unbelievable. Over the last thirty-six years, I've seen a lot of amazing things, and that was one right up near the top.

It wasn't all trauma, though. Some funny stuff happened, too. For instance, there was this lady who came in after breast augmentation surgery. When she first came in, she was still a little nauseated, and I gave her some pain meds and put a cool cloth on her neck to help her with that, and she dozed off. When she woke back up, the cloth slipped off her neck and fell down a few inches. At that point, she sat straight up on the stretcher, looked down at where the cloth had fallen, yanked up her gown, and yelled, right in front of about eighteen other patients, "I've got boobs." Then she turned to me and fired off a string of questions:

"Are they pointed in the same direction?"

"Are they the same size?"

"Do they look level?"

I was bright red, and I could barely answer her. Everybody else was in hysterics, staring at the two of us. Finally I said, "They're fine," and covered her back up.

I love taking care of patients. It might sound funny, but I love the fact that I'm actually helping them. It's the paperwork and the other crap that might eventually drive me away from it. If you were to ask me, "Should I become a nurse?" I would say, "Yes," with no hesitation, but I would recommend being selective about the area you choose.

There are good areas of nursing, but there are some where they'll just work you to death. A lot of hospitals right now want their nurses to work longer hours for less money. Med-surg floor is a killer. Orthopedics floor, they'll break your back. L&D is still okay, but then you set yourself up for liability. A lot of nurses go into that because they want to take care of the babies. I've delivered thirty-three babies in the backs of speeding ambulances, and I don't need to do that anymore.

I would look for work on a specialty unit, like maybe urology or nephrology. That area can really push you. A regular medical floor would be fine, too. Pulmonology would be good as well – you get consistent patients, with usually consistent problems. If you're an adrenaline junkie, the ER or PACU will punch your ticket and, if you can stand up for long hours at a time, you'll be okay.

That's why I like recovery: I would watch the surgery, but then I would go back out and sit down and wait for them to bring me the patient. In a PACU, you may be getting a real critical case and you'll run your butt off for a couple of hours, but you can send them away when they're stable. And then you might get a nice, easy case – someone with an appendectomy, maybe. You give them a few drugs, keep them about thirty minutes, and you send them to a floor. They're happy, and you're happy.

My brother graduated from nursing school two years ago. The day after he graduated, he turned fifty. He says the reason he went into nursing was that he saw what I did and he wanted to do the same thing. He loves it. He said there's something about it, when you're standing there and you're taking care of someone, especially in a critical-care area.

If I could just take care of patients, I'd do it all day long. I really trust in my abilities. God put me here to do this, and this is what I love to do. You can become a nurse for a lot of reasons but, for me, I sincerely believe that it's a calling. What I also love about nursing is the realization, at the end of the day, that you've done all that you could do for someone. That patient's family might see you out on the street, and they'll come up and hug you for taking good care of their mama, or their daddy, or their kid. They'll say, "Thank you," and they'll look straight into your eyes, and you'll see that they really mean it. That's what nursing is about. That's your true payment.

Of course, you can make a lot more money doing other jobs. For instance, you can make big money shooting explosives. In 1969, I was making twenty-five dollars an hour working for a construction company, blowing rock. If somebody needed a barn taken down, or a silo, we'd demolish them. Somebody wanted his land cleared, we'd run detonation cord around it and take everything down. That job let me buy a brand-new 1969 Mustang when I graduated from high school. I paid cash, $2800. It had American mags, white oval tires, four on the floor, a big breather on it. Sad to say, but I blew it up on I-20 one night. I was about two-and-a-quarter car lengths ahead of a Z-28 Camaro, and I slung a rod and spewed motor parts all over I-20. I cried a lot that day.

MELINDA CASSON

About me, abridged version: I worked in a small hospital in Oswego, New York, right out of LPN school, then moved to Pennsylvania. Worked in a family practice office there for two years, broke up, moved back to Oswego. I temped for two years in the Syracuse area, then got a job with a county-based home care agency. Worked there nine years. Now I work in wound care and hyperbaric medicine.

I don't think that everybody is necessarily cut out for wound care. There can be a bit of the gross factor to it. All nurses have to be able to deal with bodily fluids to a certain extent, but wound care can be extra smelly and slimy. In one case, I've had my hand inside somebody's chest cavity while they were awake and talking to me. In another, it was open-heart surgery gone awry, where the sternum didn't heal back together and everything was partway open.

Even the doctor was freaked out when we said, "We don't really like how this wound looks, but can you measure the depth for us? We don't feel comfortable putting a q-tip in there." She slid her fingers inside and said, "I can feel her heart beating against my fingertips." The wound wasn't wide open. You couldn't watch the heart beating. You could fit your fingers in there, but not your whole hand. I have no idea how they could survive when the heart is exposed to the open air like that. That's not supposed to happen.

Then there's gangrene, and there are maggots sometimes, and people don't always know they're there. I'd like to blame that on poor vision, but I think it's more often poor hygiene. All it takes is one fly to land and lay its beastly little eggs, and maggots love dead tissue. You know, some places use medical-grade maggots to clean wounds. We don't. Our doctors can work quickly and effectively remove dead tissue with a scalpel. That's much quicker than using medical maggots to do it. But these aren't the medical maggots I'm talking about: these are the fly-that-was-buzzing-around-your-house-and-landed-on-your-wound kinds of maggots.

Now remember, to be fair, when you have a wound that has so much dead tissue that there are maggots present, then the patient's nerve endings have died, too. They may not feel the movement. One time that happened to me. It was with a patient who lived at home, and the family member was the caregiver. Another time, it was actually a patient in a nursing home, and maggots were swarming around her toes under the dressing. The nurse that was caring for her knew I had maggot expertise. Well, I was in the hallway, and this nurse came to the patient's door and said, "Melinda? I need your help in this room." I could tell from her pale look and the tone of her voice, that it had to be maggots. I grabbed up the tools that we needed, went in and, sure enough, the wound was buzzing with them.

You have to drown them in betadine. It will kill them, but if they hit the floor they'll move really fast, especially on carpeting. Luckily, we don't have carpeting in our center. You can freeze them with ethyl chloride, which is a spray that we use for anesthetizing things rapidly, and then you drown them in the betadine. You get used to them but, I have to admit, after that first experience in home care I didn't eat meat for several weeks.

I work in a wound-care and hyperbaric-medicine center. We're a partnership between St Joseph's Hospital Health Center in Syracuse, New York, and Healogics, which is a national company that partners with hospitals to open and run these specialized centers. The job, quite literally, fell into my lap.

I had been working for a county health department home-care agency for nine years, and I had certainly seen my share of wounds. A big part of home care is changing people's bandages and using Wound V.A.C., which is a negative-pressure wound-therapy system where you actually inject a kind of porous foam into the wound. Then you seal it with something similar to sticky plastic wrap and hook a hose up under the dressing. That hose attaches to a machine that's a little larger than a fanny pack, and that's the suction unit. It removes the pus and drainage from the wound, and it decreases the risk of infection.

One of our home-care patients was a real problem. He was a pot-stirrer, playing one set of nurses against the other. Other patients told us he would do similar things at meals-on-wheels senior lunch sites. So finally we decided to put the wound-care nurses and the home-care nurses and that troublesome patient all in the same room at the wound-care center. Inadvertently, I benefited from that because I got to stay at the center for half a day, meeting people and observing the way they worked. The clinical coordinator there also became aware that I was an LPN and, when a position opened up, she encouraged me to apply for it. I ended up winning that job, and I've been lucky enough to be here for the last six years.

My mom was an LPN, too. My dad was an electrician. Sometimes he had to travel out of town for work, but he did what had to be done. He died when I was in elementary school, the summer before I started fifth grade in 1982. This was in Oswego, New York. He was a Vietnam veteran who was exposed to Agent Orange. He had returned home unaware that the chemicals were already changing his body in 1970. About ten years later, he developed a lung cancer that, after his death, was finally attributed to his exposure. It was a quick transition: from diagnosis to death, it was only eight months. After that, my mom got a job as a teacher's aide in the same elementary school that I went to, a half block from where we lived. That worked well. The hours and vacations were the same.

When I started eighth grade, my mom went back to school. She enrolled in the Oswego County BOCES School of Practical Nursing. She would be studying at the dining room table with some friends from her school, and I'd be in the living room, supposedly doing my homework. Secretly, though, I was listening to them discuss anatomy or circulation or some other subject they were studying. I was intrigued by what my mom was learning, and I absorbed some of it by osmosis.

In high school, I did well in all my subjects and was a high-honors graduate in 1992. But financial aid didn't pan out for me, so I couldn't go to college. I was working at Friendly's during my senior year in high school, so I just stayed working there. Then there was an ad in the paper for a nurse's aide training class at a nursing home, and I thought, That sounds like a good way to get my feet wet and to decide whether nursing is what I want to do. By that point, part of me definitely wanted to be a nurse, but I wasn't 100 percent positive about it. So I took the training class and worked as a nurse's aide. While I was doing that, I went to school and got my LPN at the same school where my mom had gone. I even had several of the same instructors she had, and that was fun for me.

I worked at Oswego Hospital for two years, and then I moved to Pennsylvania with the love of my life at the time. I worked in a family-practice office down there. Well, the love of my life broke up with me, and I had no idea where I was going to go. The day after that, I received a phone call from one of my mother's coworkers, telling me my mother had suffered a massive heart attack. Two life-altering events within a forty-eight-hour time frame was more than enough for me.

Luckily, my mom was at work when it happened. It was a night when the hospital was overstaffed, and it was fate that she had not gone home. Because she had a rental property, my mom had said to her supervisor, "I wouldn't mind leaving. I've got some stuff I need to do on the apartment. Somebody's coming to look at it in the morning." By that point, she had become a registered nurse, and her supervisor needed to keep an extra RN on for mandated staffing reasons. So he let one of the LPNs go home, and my mom stayed there. If she had left, she would have died that night. Not only was she at work in the hospital, but she was also downstairs in the cafeteria, which is right next to their ER.

So I flew home on an emergency plane fare and took care of her during her recuperation from open-heart surgery. I also tried to recuperate emotionally from the loss of my relationship. Eventually, I flew to Pennsylvania, packed up all my belongings, and drove back home to central New York. After that, I got a job through a temporary agency in Syracuse, working sometimes as a nurse and sometimes as a receptionist for several medical practices in the area. I wanted something more consistent, but most of the jobs I ended up with were receptionist positions, for lesser pay, and I hadn't become a nurse to work as a receptionist. When the job with the county home health care agency appeared in the paper, I applied for that. They were hiring six LPNs at that point, and I was one of the six.

I worked there for nine years, until I came here to St. Joseph's Center for Wound Care and Hyperbaric Medicine in June 2006. Three months later, on Labor Day weekend in 2006, my mother had a hemorrhagic stroke: she had an aneurysm that burst. She was in the hospital for three weeks before she passed away, and soon after that I went back to school to become an RN. I'm not sure, but I think maybe it was my way of honoring my mom and holding onto what she was.

I love my job now. My shift starts at 7:30 a.m., and my first patient arrives at 7:45. I get here, clock in, and boot up the computer in my room. Once a chart goes up on the rack, I bring the patient into the room and take the dressing off. I ask how the pain level is, and if there have been any medication changes since the last visit. Since most of our patients are here every week, I'll usually ask how the week's been. If it's the first week after Easter, for example, I'll ask, "How was your Easter? Did you go to somebody's house?" Those kinds of innocuous questions have a distinct purpose: you find out a lot by chitchat. Often, you can discover essential information that patients don't think of as important that way.

After the dressing is off, I measure the wound. Typically, the wound is going to need to be debrided, which means that the slimy residue has to be cleaned off with a scalpel by the doctor. So I'll pour some liquid lidocaine on a piece of gauze and anesthetize the wound site. We like to make it comfortable for our patients, or they resist coming back. Then I get some papers signed and give the doctor an update on the patient: "This is so-and-so. He's got that wound on his ankle. His pain's better, and he's finishing up with his antibiotics. The wound looks better. Pain is minimal."

Variations on that process occur throughout the day. There are different types of wounds, of course, so there are different procedures that we perform, but we don't take anything lightly. We consider all wounds to be potentially serious. Any non-healing wound can be a ticking timebomb. The skin is the body's first line of defense against infection, and any time you have a break, that's an open doorway for bacteria. We're not sterile human beings, no matter what germophobes would like to think. That includes me: you wouldn't believe how many times a day I wash my hands and use hand sanitizer.

To illustrate how quickly wounds can turn threatening: we had a patient recently who was doing quite well, and we applied an Apligraf.

The very next day, his wife called and told us he had suddenly started running a fever and had chills. So he came back in, and we sent him to the ER because his foot had gotten that bad, that quickly. It wasn't a reaction to the Apligraf. His circulation in that foot wasn't good to start with, and infection had damaged his bones. He's actually had part of the foot amputated, and they took quite a bit of that damaged bone out. But apparently the infection had returned.

An Apligraf is a synthetic skin graft that comes in a little petri dish. We have to order each one specifically. The Apligraf is shipped at ambient temperature – it doesn't have to be refrigerated or frozen. It has cooling gel packs in with it, so that the temperature doesn't go too high, especially in the hot months. The other types of grafts that we use, which are cadaver skin, are cryo-preserved, so they're shipped with dry ice. The cadaver skin grafts are four by four, four by eight, and four by sixteen centimeters, so they're small. But they're meshed, and they stretch. The Apligraf is a round piece, and I'll guesstimate that it's maybe five or six centimeters in diameter, maybe the size of the bottom of a styrofoam coffee cup. And Apligrafs are uniform – they only come in the one size – so occasionally we have to order more than one piece for a wound. If it's an irregularly shaped wound, the Apligraf can be cut to fit.

We use a lab-cultured skin graft. You don't want to try a split-thickness skin graft and extract a piece of skin from a patient's leg, because you've already got someone who can't heal well. Why would you want to create another wound when they can't even heal their existing wound? When you do a skin graft and take the skin from the patient, the donor site is extremely painful. It's so shallow. All the nerve endings are right there near the surface. Why inflict terrible pain on a patient when you've got a product grown in a lab that works so well?

Apligrafs aren't rejected and, quite honestly, they're easier to deal with. Cadaver skin is frozen, so you've got to thaw it, and you can't start doing that until you have the patient in the room. You don't want to start thawing it and then find out the patient has an infection. Cadaver grafts are expensive, and you don't want to waste them. The Apligraf doesn't have all the things that human skin has, but it does contain growth factors and cells, and it's been approved by the FDA for diabetic foot ulcers, which are probably the wounds we see most.

Diabetics are prone to wounds on their feet because diabetes affects circulation – not just the big arteries that can be surgically repaired or bypassed or ballooned clear, but also the little ones that feed the skin. You can't fix the little ones, and that increases their risk of sustaining wounds. Plus, over time, diabetes also damages the nerves, so patients tend to feel numb. You or I may wear a pair of shoes that may not fit right, and we're going to know that pretty quickly because our feet will hurt. Diabetics, because they lack the normal pain sensation, can walk until they've got a wound down to the bone and not even realize it. Then they take those shoes off and are shocked when they're filled with blood.

I've loved every minute of this job I have now, and I love wound care. We have a really great team – the nurses, the secretaries, and the doctors – and we all care very much about our patients. But any nurse who tells you that she doesn't have horrible days from time to time is lying. I don't go to work thinking, Hey, I'm going to save somebody's life today. I'm going to heal somebody. How pompous is that? You know, there are days where you're either burnt out with your patient load, or with your coworkers, or with something, and you go home, practicing the lines, "Would you like fries with that? Would you like to supersize that?" And that feeling may last a couple of days, but you stick with what you do, and it swings back around again. I'm my mom's daughter. I'm a nurse genetically. If something is broken, I'll try to help fix it.

It may sound odd, but I do also love some of the grossness in this job. I don't know why. I think you've got to have a sense of humor to be a nurse, but to be a wound-care nurse, you'd better have a truly bizarre sense of humor. Gallows humor is life-sustaining for us. Jokes keep us sane. Our office is unique in that we're all a bit twisted, and none of us is easily offended. Some of our lunchtime conversations would probably make the average person's hair fall out. We can eat our food and talk about the patient's wound that we saw before lunch – how bad it smelled and how the patient pooped all over while we were doing the dressing. We can talk that way and not miss a bite, I swear. To somebody who doesn't understand the occupation, though, our humor could probably sound crass.

I also really like teaching patients and having to direct my teaching to their level of comprehension. You've got to adjust your vocabulary and explain clearly what their problem is and how they have to take care of it. Some patients want to know all the things they can do to help themselves. Others want to know less. So you've got to learn a lot about your patients to make sure they can learn from you.

I do have some things that make me sad, of course. We've had patients whose wounds were caused by cancer. Sometimes the patients come to us already aware of that, but many times we're the ones who do the biopsy, diagnose it, and have to tell them they have it. Those are the worst, because when they have a wound and come to the wound specialist, they think they're going to be fixed. And we have to tell them, "We're sorry, but that's cancer, and you need to have surgery."

I felt terrible for this one patient who had melanoma. She suffered with lumps that kept growing from her body, bursting open and ulcerating. And they smelled awful – that cancer-wound smell which is immediately stomach-turning. The patient knew what she had, and she could see that more and more were popping out. She would be looking down at her body as her wound was being changed and say, "Oh, look, there's another new one. That wasn't open yesterday, but today it's draining. Gosh, that smells terrible." It wasn't bad enough that she had a cancer that would ultimately kill her, but she had to stink like death all the way through it and be aware of that.

Sometimes you have to just remember the funny things to get through. I can remember when I was in the nurse's aide class in the nursing home, there was one little old lady sitting in a rocking chair, wearing her flowered house dress. She was knitting, and she looked up at us all, proud as could be, and announced that she was knitting an African. I can still picture her in my head, and I use that when I need to laugh.

DR. DANETTE WOOD

Over the last twenty-seven years as a registered nurse, I have cared for thousands of patients at their bedside. In addition, as an educator for eighteen years, I have watched more than 1000 of my nursing students graduate with their baccalaureate in nursing degrees and enter the workforce. In 2003, I was awarded Georgia Southern University's Excellence in Teaching Award.

When we were very young, my twin sister and I invented our own kind of twinning language, and we communicated with each other that way. But Denise and I were the last two kids in the family, and Mama was too busy with the other four. So it took a while for her to figure our language out.

Mama taught all of us that we would be college graduates, and so that was simply the expectation. But I didn't find out, until she gave us our history just before she died, that she was never really talking to me. Because I couldn't talk to her, she didn't realize I was there. That's quite a common thing with stammerers – it's almost like we don't exist. I was never supposed to be able to be educated. I was classified as an imbecile because I didn't talk. That was the reason they kept me out of public school. That's quite normal, if you look at the research. So I never realized that I was supposed to be dependent and be taken care of and not succeed.

My mother put me in private Catholic school because she thought the nuns would love me even though, at that time, educators felt that the inability to communicate verbally equated with an inability to learn. Although no one told me I could not learn, I was amazed when I did learn. And I knew from the second grade, when Sister Ann introduced me to the wonderment of knowledge, that I wanted to follow her example – I wanted to teach. It never occurred to me that, without a voice, I probably wouldn't be able to do it.

I don't remember a lot of my childhood because I think I blocked it out, but my twin provided some information. I do remember that she acted as my voice. I actually stammered over 80 percent of my syllables, so that meant I could not clearly articulate a two-syllable word. I used to slide a vowel sound ahead of a word to help me say it. If I did try to speak, what came out sounded like gibberish. I can understand why others thought I was an imbecile if that was the only kind of communication I was able to make. Nobody could understand me except my twin sister. Denise would take over and speak for me and, even if I didn't say a word, she intuited what I wanted to say. She was so close to me that she could complete my sentences and, to this day, I can complete hers. She's in Florida now, and we talk just about every other day. It's almost like we're symbiotic.

Because I made myself work so hard, I graduated from high school with the third-highest GPA in my class. I was still determined to be a teacher, so I tried to get into a public teaching college. This was in 1972, and college was a privilege at that time. The only disabled individuals who got any breaks were the soldiers, because the disability act at that time only applied to returning GIs. The public didn't get an opportunity to benefit from the public money until the Rehabilitation Act was passed in September 1973. So when I interviewed at public colleges, they saw I couldn't communicate properly and they wouldn't accept my application.

At that time, the idea was that public education used public funds – tax dollars – and from a legislative viewpoint, you couldn't expend public funds on individuals who might not prove profitable for society. It wasn't considered discrimination. It was seen as a political responsibility not to waste the public's money. Deaf people got their opportunities starting in the early 1900s, when schools for the deaf were started, but it was different with me. I could hear and I could make sounds, but I couldn't talk. There weren't specific schools for stammerers.

I was finally accepted into a private college where the faculty advised me to pursue art. After completing my associate's degree in art, I got married and had a daughter, Christina. When she was three, I found a job as an unskilled laborer in a factory. I was an introvert, and I honestly don't know, if I hadn't learned to speak, whether I'd still be alive. I really don't. It was a very discouraging life. I had thoughts of suicide, but

Christina kept me going. I had a responsibility to her. I was also Catholic, and that instilled a reverence for life as well. My life back then wasn't very pleasant. I was extremely isolated, and I had an abusive husband, too, so that hindered everything. After he left us, I came close to killing myself, but I just couldn't, because I thought, *I am a woman, and I am a mother, and Christina needs me.*

Everybody has troubles to face, of course. My grandma raised ten children on her own. Her husband killed himself because he had an incurable disease, and her smallest child was not even a year old at the time. And I came up from a family where my dad had taken off when my mom was twenty-eight, and that was before she carried us twins home from the hospital. We asked her, when we talked to her about the family history, why she didn't kill herself, and she said, "Well, I thought about it, but I couldn't find anybody who would take all six kids, and I wasn't going to split my family up. So I had to stick around and support you." She had two jobs, because incomes for women at that time were really low. But she said it was her responsibility, and her choice, and she wasn't about to rely on charity.

So I set my heart on being a nurse rather than a teacher. I still had to get an education, because I knew that working in a factory wouldn't satisfy me. It wasn't enough. However, when I applied to the local practical-nursing program, I discovered that they didn't want me, either. However, that same year, there was a student who had taken a school to court under the Rehabilitation Act, and all of the schools were watching the case. The first court said that a disabled student did not qualify, and the second court threw it back because of a procedural error. So it was up before the Supreme Court. I applied to that school at the very time a decision was being considered. School officials finally informed me that they had to allow me into their nursing school, though, because the Rehabilitation Act of 1973 had recently been signed into law. However, they did counsel me that I would never get a job because I couldn't communicate properly.

It was quite a hostile environment. They thought I was taking the place of a student who could profit from the education and succeed. I even had to sign a statement saying that I understood that I would never be able to get a job. Just my being there made them angry, and they allowed the other students to tease me. I got even by messing up the grade curve. I wasn't an imbecile after all. I was doing better than most of the other students, and – surprise, surprise – out of the class of forty-three students, only fourteen of us graduated. I was number two. I not only graduated near the top of my class, I also got a job almost right away.

Now it turned out that if I had applied a year earlier, before the Rehab Act was passed, I wouldn't have gotten in. If I had applied a year later, I wouldn't have gotten in, either, because the Supreme Court upheld the first court's decision. I guess I was in the right place at the right time for once.

As a nurse, I found my purpose and I loved it. To communicate at the hospital, I would write things down, because I still was extremely disfluent. My patients loved me because I listened to them, and that was unique. And it was at the hospital that I actually saw a television program about Annie Glenn, John Glenn's wife, who also had a horrible stammer. That's how I found out about Hollins, which was the place that I say "opened my mouth."

Now when I say Hollins, I mean the Hollins Speech Institute, which was affiliated with Hollins College. It was amazing. I actually stayed there for a whole month. They taught me how to breathe and how to control the articulators – which means that I still had the stammer, but I could control it most of the time. In thirty days, I learned a technique that let me speak almost normally. The words came out slowly, and my speech was a monotone, but I was speaking.

At the time, it was extremely expensive. It cost me six weeks of my gross income. But it was awesome. To this day, I go back occasionally and go through the training program all over again just to keep up the skills. I am still a stammerer and I wonder, most of the time, whether I will speak clearly in particular instances. It's been a lot of hard work, and far too much money, because a chronic disorder is pay-as-you-go. It's not under any insurance plan, but it's all been worth it. I haven't got good penmanship, and I don't write real fast, and I can't type too well.

But learning to speak without stammering opened up my life. I mean, it literally started a new life for me when I was twenty-six years old.

The first time I called my mother on the telephone, she got angry and blamed it on my sister. She said, "That's not funny, Denise." And I said, "I'm not Denise." Even though I hadn't spoken a lot, when I didn't stammer I sounded just like my twin sister. I couldn't believe it: I could finally speak on the phone for the first time in my life, and my seven-year-old daughter no longer had to order for me when we ate at a restaurant.

During my first six years as a nurse, I worked all over. I finally landed in an ICU but, as an LPN, you are limited. You can't advance. However, I wanted to achieve more as a nurse and decided to pursue my RN. I had looked at other schools, and the area I lived in had a college in it. I did have the degree in art that I had earned at art school, and I had completed all my core courses, but that college wanted me to start all over. I looked at the courses and thought, *Well, I can handle everything except college math again.*

Then someone told me I should talk to a nurse on another floor, because she was going to a college that accepted your course work from other places. It was distance learning, and I thought, *Maybe I could do that. I'm a disciplined person.* But my speech was not perfect, and I remembered the obstacles that educators had put before me when I had applied to college in the past.

But Regents College was different. They didn't interview the candidates in person so they would never know that I was not perfectly articulate. They offered a flexible schedule where the students planned their own programs, and that enabled me to continue to work full time. And since my previous degree was from an accredited college, they accepted my past courses to finish off the core curriculum. I completed college proficiency exams to satisfy the prerequisite sciences that I didn't have. Since I couldn't afford to buy the books, I checked them out of the local college library and then scheduled my finals. Within a year, I had completed the courses and clinical proficiency exam to complete the associate's degree in nursing. I also scheduled and passed my nursing licensure exam on the first attempt.

After that, I immediately started my BSN, although I could take it slower since I was now earning an RN's salary and was able to afford to buy the books. In the back of my mind, I still dreamed of teaching, but I wasn't ready. Even though Hollins had given me fluency, it remained an unstable fluency: If I was fatigued, it was hard to control my speech, and I had little confidence. I would get into stressful situations and lose my ability to use the techniques I had learned. For instance, I couldn't speak under pressure. Sometimes I could speak as clear as a bell, but if I had to stand up in a group, it became much harder. Maybe that was the reason why I pushed it and wanted to become a teacher – once again, to prove to myself I could accomplish it. I've only ever been satisfied with achievement, because I shouldn't have been able to do much of what I've done.

But I did love working in the ICU. If it was a little slow in my unit, I was able to connect with the patients' families. And I was good with death. I know that sounds awful, but if anybody who was dying came in, I would get them assigned to me, because I could talk to their families and help them through it. New nurses have real difficulty with that aspect. It takes a while to understand how to handle death.

What I love about nursing is that it offers me the chance to help patients who are often in helpless situations. I've had patients ask me, "Am I going to die?" and I've thought, Yeah, there isn't anything I can do, though I wouldn't ever say that to them. I had one patient look at me, and he was really scared. "Am I dying?" he asked, and I stuck my hand on my hip and said, "Absolutely not. I'm here. And it's too much paperwork." So he laughed, and said, "Well, if you can crack jokes, maybe I won't die." You know what? He didn't. It was amazing. You have to calm patients down. Anxiety causes all sorts of chemicals to swirl around in their bodies, and that will make them get worse.

When I completed my BSN, I applied to Georgia Southern University and entered their masters of science in nursing program. Since many of the instructors there had worked with me in area hospitals, I had no difficulty getting accepted into the program. When I completed my MSN at Georgia Southern, while I was working full time in my hospital job, I was still thinking about trying to teach, but it was scary. Then an unexpected opportunity came my way.

At the local tech school, one of the teachers left two days before the start of classes because of a family emergency. The school was desperate and they didn't care if I stood on my head in the corner and spat nickels. I had my MSN, and they hired me as a temporary teacher to teach the anatomy and physiology course. I thought, They have to have somebody, so I'll give it a try. Well, the students loved how I taught, because I could reduce difficult concepts to an easy-to-understand level. Even though I still stammered off and on, I was able to connect with the students and help them understand the subject. They loved me. I was guiding the students, and the students were learning. I was hooked.

After I completed temporary positions as adjunct faculty for two of the local technical nursing programs, Georgia Southern University hired me as a temporary instructor in their nursing program. Over the next several years, I worked full time as an educator and part-time as an ICU nurse at the local hospital. In 1999, I graduated with my doctorate in education degree and became an assistant professor of nursing. This was twenty-seven years after being refused entry into a public teacher education program.

In the first class of each new semester, I always stand up and say, "I have a little stammer." If I don't explain it ahead of time, I always have it in my head that the audience won't really know what's wrong. They won't hear my presentation because they'll be thinking, *What is wrong with that individual?* Even when I have spoken in different places across the country – because I'm not always positive if it will come out clearly or if I will stammer – I always start off by explaining that I have a slight stammer. I also explain that it really annoys me because it slows me down.

A few years ago, my school wanted to give me a prestigious award, and I almost refused it, because it required that I speak in front of the student body and the faculty. We had 600 teachers at that time and I thought, *Oh, my God, I can't do that. I can't speak in public.* Then I realized two things: many of the faculty might be too busy to attend, and the award came with a significant monetary gift. I wanted that, of course, but I also wanted to be acknowledged as an excellent teacher. I reassured myself by thinking, *Nobody will come.*

But the day I spoke, the chair of my department was there, and I said, "Now, Jean, get out of here. You make me nervous. Come on, Jean, please leave." And she wouldn't. Then the deans came, and I said, "Come on. Get out of here. This is too much pressure." And they laughed. They really didn't believe that they made me nervous, and they didn't know the anxiety could make me stammer. But I was horribly nervous, and I was afraid that I was going to ruin everything and lose my job. I thought, *Why in the world did they come?* They weren't supposed to be there. They never came to those events.

Then the president of the university showed up, and that's something which had only happened a few times. *Oh, Christ,* I thought, *I really will lose my job now. Academia is so stuffy.* So I got up, and the first thing that came out of my mouth was, "You guys are an intimidating audience. I have a slight stammer, so this could be a problem." And they all laughed, thank goodness. So I spoke for an hour and a half. I wasn't supposed to, but nobody dared stop me. I thought, *Well, if I'm going to lose my job, I'm going out with a bang.* I figured if I could do that and not lose my job, well, I could do anything.

I think about some of the struggles I have had, and some of the opportunities, and that frames how I think about my own students. I look at students who have learning disabilities, and I wonder, *Can they do this?* And by golly, they do, and they surprise every one of us. I don't let myself feel my natural empathy for them. I have to challenge that and tell them to quit complaining and figure out how they can succeed. I am the hardest on them, because I don't let them say, "Poor me." I tell them, "Let's not fail. Let's go ahead and succeed."

And it's awesome, because they almost always out-do your expectations, and they do succeed, and I think, *They did it, and I didn't really think it was possible. And school is so hard now.* I'm glad I'm not a student today. I'm glad I did it a long time ago, when we didn't have blood-sugar machines and technology. I was lucky. I stretched my education out over twenty years, and that gave me the opportunity to savor learning and experience the wonder of gaining knowledge.

JODY BEDARD

I received my associate's degree in nursing in 2008, and I was licensed as a registered nurse in Maryland in 2009. On active duty with the Navy, I am currently assigned as a nurse corps officer in the traumatic brain injury ward at Walter Reed National Medical Center in Bethesda. Before receiving my nursing degree, I had served as a Navy corpsman for approximately fifteen years. During that time, I had multiple deployments as a combat corpsman with both Navy and Marine Corps units serving in the Persian Gulf, Kuwait, Iraq, Somalia, Rwanda, Guam, and in New Orleans for Hurricane Katrina.

I live in Maryland, but in 2007, before I had my nursing license, I was deployed to Iraq. While I was there, I had to call back home. Now mind you, this phone conversation was at 8 o'clock at night for me and 8 o'clock in the morning for them, and we took some sniper fire while I was talking. The lady on the other end of the phone worked for the Maryland State Board of Nursing, and she was kind of freaking out. "Oh my God, is that gunfire in the background?" she asked.

Maryland was in the middle of deciding to pull the plug on allowing Excelsior students to become licensed here. The deans and directors of the state's traditional nursing programs weren't crazy about Excelsior's competency-based examinations, and they pressured the state nursing board to set one final date for their graduates to be eligible to take the NCLEX, the licensure exam. I was in Iraq at the time, and I called to say all I had left to complete were my clinicals, but I needed more time. "What is that noise?" she asked again.

"Yeah, those are gunshots. I'm in the middle of a combat zone," I told her.

"Put the phone down," she hollered.

"Lady," I said, "you don't know how hard it's been for me to get a hold of you. I'm not putting the phone down. I'm calling to tell you that I can get this done, but not until I get back. I need a little more time."

When I returned, I testified before the Maryland State Senate about the Excelsior program. The commander of my hospital, who went on to become the Navy Surgeon General, had written a letter on my behalf, saying essentially, "Look, this guy should be allowed to get his license. This is what he did in Iraq."

My point was, if I'm only able to go to school in this manner – studying in my hooch, hearing rifle fire, and feeling bullets hit the walls – then I should be able to go and take these tests whenever I get back. Service to my country should be worth that much consideration. There are many other corpsmen and medics who are trying to graduate and become nurses, too. Maybe their personal stories are slightly different than mine but, basically, the principle is the same: they know the information, they have the skills, and they use both in combat settings every single day. Do they really need to be sitting in a classroom to prove they're competent as nurses? Should we be denied our licenses because we learned in a different way? To me, this is like a no-brainer. But as of right now, I'm the last Excelsior nursing student who has gotten licensed in the state of Maryland.

I was in Iraq that last time from May 2007 until March 2008. Initially I was in Habbaniya, but once they found out I was in nursing school and was about the next best thing to having a doctor, they sent me out by myself with a special ops team. We were stationed in a couple of houses right along the Euphrates River. The battalion aid station was essentially a one-story house with a small room upstairs that had four walls and no windows. That's where I was working, right smack dab in the middle of freakin' IED alley.

I spent practically every waking minute with the medics over there, and we did have insurgents who had infiltrated the Iraqi battalion stationed with us. So there was no way to know who those people were. We had to screen the entire battalion, and some people popped with fingerprints. One of them – a medic I had worked with and with whom I had been alone, seeing patients, more times than I could count – had his fingerprints identified on a fragment of an IED that had killed a Navy SEAL. It wasn't the safest place, and I just had to trust that I would be okay.

We were in charge of the only two bridges between Ramadi and Fallujah. Our primary mission was to protect those bridges. Our secondary mission was to train the special forces Iraqi army battalion, so I really made an effort to focus on their health. I was responsible for taking care of about 900 Iraqi soldiers, as well as our special ops guys.

Plus, there were about 6,000 civilians in the local population and, by default, I became a stand-in for their town doctor. I was also doing sick call with the regular Marines, and most of my guys were fine. I had to do immunizations and had to check for tuberculosis because a couple of the Iraqis had shown up with active TB. I was doing everything I could to make sure that everybody was staying in one piece and healthy.

I was able to cut down substantially on the food-borne illnesses the battalion suffered. In the Middle East, they don't have the kinds of toilets we do at home. They just have a hole in the ground, that's it, and they had a few of these holes way too close to where they were preparing their food. I had to tell them, "You've got to move these. Just watch. See the flies over there? See the guy over here cooking? Watch how the flies go back and forth between the two places." So it took them a while, but they finally figured out what I was talking about. Then they brought in some cutting boards and clean tables. A lot of recommendations I made they acted on very quickly, and the food-borne illnesses went from ten cases a week to practically none.

We were taking sniper fire every now and then. In our first few days there, an IED exploded right outside the compound. One of the Iraqi police officers was killed in that blast. On another occasion, some Iraqi policemen were poking at an IED, rather than calling for help or leaving it alone. That one exploded also, killing one and injuring two more. One of them came in with shrapnel all over him.

In a third incident, two Iraqi police trucks were traveling down the road, and a guy in the back of one wanted to switch vehicles. So as these trucks were bouncing along a crappy, IED-bombed road, he tried jumping from one truck into the other as they drove side by side, but he didn't make it. When he fell, he sustained this two-inch, perfectly-round skull fracture on the left side of his head. Now I had seen a skull fracture before, but I hadn't seen one with the indentation protruding into the brain like that, and certainly not one where the guy was still talking.

"Oh my God," I said. "I need to get this guy out of here." Well, I couldn't send him to the American shock trauma platoon, where they did surgery, because he wasn't really Iraqi police – he was one of the

Neighborhood Watch guys. Then his pupils started to change a little bit, and I told the Iraqi medics, "You guys have to do something. If we're going to save him, you've got to get him somewhere right now." So I sacrificed one of our backboards, and they took him into Fallujah. They didn't have much of a hospital there, but it was something.

A few weeks after that, there was an incident in which a thirteen-year-old girl fell into the fire that her family constantly burned in front of their house. They wanted her to live, so they didn't take her to the town "medic." They brought her to me. She had mostly second-degree and some third-degree burns, basically from her neck to her toes. I used a lot of the fire gel pack that we have – a sterile bandage that you can cover wounds with – and I started her on antibiotics and pain medications. I did what I could. I also sent an e-mail back to the UCSD Burn Center and asked them what I needed to be looking for in prolonged treatment. If I were to save her, I needed to know exactly what I was doing. Fortunately, a Navy surgeon who was a burn specialist e-mailed back and gave me some good instructions.

It was too dangerous for her to keep coming back to the compound, so I went to her home. We'd go out on combat foot patrol, and I'd bring my medical gear, my rifle, my shotgun, and pistol. We were doing the foot patrol for security, but we would swing by the house where she lived so I could change her dressing and monitor her condition.

She survived. She definitely had some scarring, but I knew I wouldn't be able to treat that. As it turned out, she was one of the nieces of the sheikh in that area, and he had a lot of influence. After she pulled through, a lot of the violence really dropped off. The IEDs that were being planted, the mortar attacks, the sniper fire we had been taking – all of it suddenly stopped. It was like somebody just turned off the switch.

Something similar happened when I was in Somalia in 1994. In Somalia, I was with 2nd Battalion 5th Marines, the most decorated battalion in the Marine Corps. They tend to be the ones you see in all the movies like *Battlefield L.A.* and *Full Metal Jacket.* They're the ones that get picked to do more: for example, the first Marine Corps unit to go into Baghdad in the invasion was 2-5. They led the whole pack.

Somalia was pretty hectic. We actually went into the country to evacuate the rest of the American forces about six months after the Blackhawk Down incident. There were a few firefights that broke out as we were trying to get everybody out of Mogadishu.

It was mostly desert there – a lot of sand with a few grasses. Not a whole lot of trees. It was really dry because we were so close to the equator, and the temperature probably hit about 120 degrees during the day. I was responsible for making sure my Marines were drinking enough water and taking their malaria medication. We had to drink a liter of water every hour just to make sure we maintained our hydration.

We weren't in downtown Mogadishu – that was about five or six miles away – so we didn't have to worry about safety every second. We had about 150 Marines, and we were inside an old police training compound that had been pretty bombed out. If you were to look at it, you'd say, "This place was definitely once a combat zone." The compound sat on some cliffs right above the beach. We were like a quick-reaction force, making sure none of the warlords came in and set up camp south of the city. We used night vision technology, and we had the advantage of seeing what was coming down the road. There was one dirt road that was going north and south along the coastline, and at night we could sit out there and watch people walk by with their camels. There were even some who had elephants.

A lot of the wounded were from other units up north. We had a few injuries but nothing too major, so I could pay some attention to the civilians in the area. There was a little tribe near us that was called the Somali Clan. You had to walk down the hill towards the beach to reach them. They were fasting when we got there, for one of their religious holidays, but after a few days, they pulled a sea turtle out of the Indian Ocean and roasted it up. The kids were walking around eating turtle meat on sticks. Well, I walked the edge of our compound area every day, and I saw that some of these kids had cuts and scrapes on them. So through an interpreter, I offered to take care of them. Then there was one kid who had an infection on his foot, and I treated him, too.

Pretty soon, the adults started coming by – elderly men, mostly, not any females – and they had bad knees, or arthritis, or maybe some old injuries. I gave them a few medications, some bandages, some Ace wraps. I remember with this one elderly guy, I wrapped up both his knees and gave him some Ibuprofen, and I had some Icy Hot that I put on his legs. The next day he had this huge smile on his face.

When one of the interpreters told him that we were going to be pulling out soon, this old guy told him that, of all the troops that had been there before, no one had ever cared enough to go into their community and help anybody. So then they actually brought me a few gifts: some beaded necklaces and that type of stuff, but one had knitted a hat out of yarn, and one of the guys had carved the Virgin Mary from a piece of wood. They were Muslim, mind you, but they knew the story of Jesus and Mary. And he had carved little angels on the bottom, too. He wasn't an artist, but the guy had really made a valiant attempt, and I knew exactly what it was when I looked at it. One of them gave me the only money he had. It was this really old Italian-minted Somali silver coin, about the size of a silver dollar, and it had a jaguar and a crescent moon on it, I remember that. For poor people, that was a lot to give.

I was touched. I hadn't known that no one else had tried to help them. For me, that was a really tough point in my life, because my marriage was falling apart, and so I had that playing in the background all the time. I was on a mission, I guess, trying to find something that might add a little good to the world.

Honestly, for me, nursing never gets boring. There's enough constant change that it doesn't feel monotonous. It isn't always just treating the patients you expect to have. For instance, the other day at Walter Reed, there was a family who came in. Their son had been severely injured by an IED in Afghanistan the week before. This was Monday afternoon, and I was trying to direct them to where they could buy some Chapstick, believe it or not. Their son had chapped lips, and they were just trying to help out in whatever small way they could.

My hands were full. I was hurrying out of there. I had my dress whites in one hand, and I held my shoes, my stethoscope, and a little notebook in the other. It would have been easier for me to tell them to go down the hallway, go left and then right – easier for me to hurry to my car to make my appointment. But they had this look on their faces, like they had never been in a hospital before, so I just walked them down to where the little store was. They were very appreciative, and they asked me why – because I have like ten rows of ribbons, and obviously I've been around for a while – "Why do you keep doing this?"

I said, "Because of kids like your son. I feel like he's my kid brother. Any of the patients here could be my brother, or my uncle, or my next-door neighbor. To me, they're all family. If I'm not giving them my all, I shouldn't be here. These kids are putting their lives on the line. You don't have to agree with war, but somebody's got to step up and fight. I can guarantee there are a lot of people who have decided it sure won't be them, and it's not going to be their kids who are doing it, either. So this is my way of honoring the ones who say they will do it."

ALICIA LEPARD

*In 1993, I earned an associate's degree.
At the time, I was working at a military
installation on Johnson Atoll, a small
island in the Pacific Ocean, where I
transitioned from being a paramedic to
an RN. After that, I couldn't stop studying
and learning. In 1998, I graduated with
my bachelor's degree and then completed
my first master's degree in 2003.
I currently have four master's degrees
in all, including an MBA in health
care. I now work full time at a clinic
in Gillette, Wyoming, specializing in
the care of people with diabetes.*

I grew up in the '70s, so I remember Johnny and Roy in *Emergency*. I still have a clipping from *Parade* magazine of the first female L.A. Fire Department paramedic, and I wanted to be a paramedic as well. In the early '70s, that's what it was all about for me. So I became an EMT in 1980 and a paramedic in 1981. I was one of the youngest paramedics when I got my license – only eighteen years old. I thought that was what I wanted to be for the rest of my life. But my dad said, "You should have a backup plan. You should go to nursing school, too." Well, I tried the traditional route during my first year of college and flunked dismally. I got a GPA of 1.8. So I dropped out of the pre-nursing track and switched over to the paramedic program. In Michigan, which is where I grew up, they offered their paramedic programs through the local colleges.

My first job was with a little service called Aarrow Ambulance, in Grand Rapids, Michigan, and they were affiliated with Bud's Ambulance. I swear that was the name of the company. I even have the patches to prove it. Bud's ran eight ambulances through the city of Grand Rapids, and that was a pretty substantial service until it got closed down. I worked a twenty-four-hour shift, 8:00 a.m. one day to 8:00 a.m. the next. Acclimating was difficult, but it was also a wild time.

I rode the ambulance in Grand Rapids until 1983, and then I went over and worked in the Detroit area for Riverside, an ambulance company associated with a funeral home in Novi, Michigan. Then I worked for Jackson EMS, in Jackson, Michigan, until about 1985. We were a lot busier there. Grand Rapids had been an upscale community, but when I started working in the Detroit area, I saw real poverty for the first time.

I can remember walking into project housing at four in the morning and being shocked at how people were living there. You would walk down the hallways and hear the babies screaming through the thin walls, and you realized there were hundreds of people shoehorned into that cramped area. And because it was 4:00 a.m. and an ambulance had shown up, everybody came out to see what all the excitement was about. One particular night, a baby had died. But as soon as people realized that, they acted like, Oh, is that all it is? Okay, back into our apartments. Ignore everybody else again.

Where I was born and raised, neighbors and friends would have rushed to comfort the family and to help out in any way they could. What I saw in the projects didn't make any sense to me at first, but it was an eye-opener. It was hard to survive there, and it took too much energy to care if another baby died. For me, that was a foreign way of life, and I had to figure out how to function in that kind of world. But I was young and excited to learn things I wish now I didn't know: that people die traumatically; that people shoot each other; that people can be unfeeling and apathetic.

On the other hand, I got to have some adventures, too. After I left Jackson, I went to work in Alaska. I had applied for the job because I had seen an ad in the back of an EMS journal. They called me for an interview, and my dad said, "If you're up there and they want to keep you, don't come home. I'll send your stuff." I arrived there on a Friday, and they said, "Yeah, we'd like to hire you." They asked me when I could start, and I answered, "Monday sounds good. Do you have a place I can stay for the weekend?" They arranged to find me a house, and I spent five years up there.

It was a great job, working for the Southern Region EMS. I got to travel the southern half of the state and teach the ambulance squads. My apartment was in Anchorage, but I would fly all over. I trained squads in Soldotna, Bethel, Dutch Harbor, and Cold Bay, among others. Most of the time, a pilot would drop me off at a village and say, "See you in a couple of weeks." When I finished the classes, I'd rest up in Anchorage for a week or two and then I'd fly out to someplace else.

I did experience some strange accommodations: in Bethel, I bunked in the fire department. In Cold Bay, I lived in one of the patient rooms in their clinic. In Dutch Harbor, I stayed in a nun's apartment because the nun, who was part of the EMS squad, was away. That was when I realized that some Catholics drank a lot of alcohol. I was sheltered – what can I say?

That job was federally funded and, after five years, the funding ran out. Again, I answered an ad in the back of an EMS journal, and I went to Las Vegas to work for what was then Mercy Ambulance Service. Now it's AMR, American Medical Response. I was a street medic, but I was also training other medics, and I was still learning myself. I was always going to school. Every place I've ever lived, I've taken a class in something or other. I've studied everything, from sign language to algebra, making sure I studied the core subjects that would be required for a college degree. Piecemeal, I just kept adding to my education.

Las Vegas was where I learned about gangs and drugs. Back then, it was the early age of what we called "ice." Now I know it was methamphetamine. I remember we got a call in the middle of the night, about 3:00 a.m., to what we thought was a suicide – a dead body in an apartment building – but nobody could find the body's head. From the evidence, it had been traumatically ripped off. A little later, we learned that somebody had used a hammer on the guy and then had thrown his head up into a tree. As daybreak arrived, and just as we were packing up to leave, one of my crew spotted it up there, and we retrieved it.

That kind of violence was pretty common in Las Vegas, more than in probably any other place I had worked. It was the days of the Bloods and the Crips and the Kings all fighting each other. Eventually, I just got used to it, but becoming callous carries consequences, too. The subsequent investigation proved that it was all over a drug deal – a four- or five-dollar difference in price or something. It was stupid and pointless. Up until then, I had just skated along the periphery of knowing about all the drugs and the culture associated with them. So that was my initiation into, "It's a big bad world here."

I remember one day, it was early morning, maybe 5:00 or 6:00 a.m. The sun was slightly up, and there had been a shooting near a schoolyard. I was treating one of the gang members who had been involved in the shooting. He had a small wound in his leg, and he was lying in the back of the ambulance, groaning loudly. I refused to start the transport to the hospital until he told me where he had ditched his gun. I was terrified that the kids coming to school in the morning would find it and we'd have a child shot accidentally. He didn't think I had enough power to wait him out, but I did. He finally told me where the gun was, and we retrieved it and gave it to the cops before we took him to the hospital. He wasn't bleeding out, but he certainly hurt, and I wouldn't give him morphine until he told us where that gun was. It was just one small thing I could do to make sure that innocent people were a little safer.

We also had a cardiac arrest in a bingo parlor, and the lady lived. She waved as we were wheeling her out of the bingo parlor and the whole slots audience got up and applauded madly. *Okay,* I thought, *that's why I do this.* For Las Vegas, that qualified as a heart-warming event.

Another day in Las Vegas, my blood sugars wouldn't rise above fifty the whole day. I've had Type 1 diabetes since I was seventeen. My mother died of diabetes at age fifty-five, and her sisters also died in their fifties of the disease. We have a long history of diabetes in my family, and I've always gotten a little annoyed about the fact that people gave me rules that wouldn't work, or couldn't offer anything that truly helped. So by the end of that particular day, I got a little nervous about going to bed. I drove to one of the emergency rooms and talked them into just keeping an eye on me. They shoved me into a corner and ignored me for six hours. They did finally check to see whether I was pregnant, and I said, "Really? That's the sum total of what you're going to do for me? Okay, this was an expensive adventure into health care. Apparently, I'm fine. I'll be going home now."

I stayed in Las Vegas until 1990, and after that I ended up on Johnston Island, out in the middle of the Pacific Ocean. I was having a hard time controlling my blood sugars out there – my A1c was 13 percent, which is horribly high. It should be below 7 percent. I went to an endocrinologist in Honolulu, and he said, "Well, you can't just pull twenty-four-hour shifts and do this kind of work. You need a controlled life in order to live with diabetes." And I remember looking at him and saying, "Are you giving me a job in your clinic so I can work nine to five? Because that's not what I do for a living."

"No," he answered, "but you're going to die of diabetes because you're not doing the right things." Then he gave me the list of whatever he thought I wasn't doing right. That was one of the starting points of what would become my career in diabetes care.

The ad I saw for that job on the island was actually in the Sunday newspaper in Las Vegas. It said, LOOKING FOR A PARAMEDIC TO GO OUT TO A REMOTE ISLAND SITE. It was an ad from Holmes and Narver Services. When I went to my interview, they said, "We want you to go work on this island. It's two miles long. It's a half mile wide. Very tropical. And oh, by the way, we're in the process of eliminating chemical weapons out there. We're going to begin destroying them on June 30. Do you want to be part of the team?"

I took all their stuff and said, "Gosh, I do want to be part of this team," and so I filled out an application, and they accepted me. I packed up my household, deposited all of it in a storage site, and I moved across the ocean. They were paying a lot of money, at that time, for a paramedic. You have to realize that I was making ten bucks an hour and trying to live on that in Las Vegas. They offered me free room and board and flights back and forth, and the chance to go out to this tropical island where the temperature was seventy degrees all the time – plus the fact that here was a whole new side of EMS. There was no backup – nothing. I would be the sole medical professional on an island eight hundred miles southwest of Hawaii. What I had were the people who were out there with me and the equipment that was right there. The whole idea of being in such a remote location fascinated me.

I showed up on April Fools Day in 1990 and plunged right in. The medical staff was responsible for the health and welfare of about twelve hundred people at any given time. We handled occupational medicine and emergency care medicine, and we were tasked, of course, with the mission of being prepared for any chemical weapons exposure. We maintained a medical clinic as well, and our main purpose there was to support six ventilator-dependent patients for twenty-four hours, if necessary. I remember I walked in there, and nobody knew how to run a ventilator. So I bought a couple of books and taught myself how to run it, and then I taught everybody else how to do it. That was how we learned to run ventilators. Thank God, we never had to use them.

Johnston Island was a pseudo-military installation. They had used it as a chemical weapons storage facility before and during World War II, and they were still trying to destroy those munitions – nerve gas and mustard agents, for example. The chemical weapons had been sitting in bunkers for so long that they were essentially rotting.

Everybody lived on one corner of the island, because the rest of it was taken up by the runway and by the burn plant. And then there was a part of the island which had been exposed to Agent Orange and plutonium missiles, and you weren't allowed to go there either. Johnson Atoll had been a Safeguard C testing site in the '60s and '70s. One of the missiles during that time had fallen over on the pad and contaminated it. The island had originally been owned by the Navy, but the Army had control of the chemical munitions. The Air Force ran the airstrip. The Coast Guard was out there on a LORAN – a long range navigation station. It was basically a military installation with government contract workers.

It probably sounds a little scary, but it was paradise. We had an outdoor movie theater, an Olympic-size swimming pool, a six-lane bowling alley, and an ocean to go play in. But we also served as the prototype facility for the destruction of chemical weapons. Our process was to burn them. They would literally open up these canisters and munitions, extract the agents, and burn them. Burn teams had to wear seal-a-meal suits with self-contained air because chemical weapons constitute one of the highest levels of hazmat. They basically employ heat to seal the suit, to make it one unit, and those guys would stay in those suits for up to an hour and a half, sweating like crazy in there. We actually did some of the first heat-stress studies for the Army with those guys, because we could test them for their dehydration before and after they would make the entries in their suits. They could easily drop seven to ten pounds, or more, during an excursion.

One day in early 1993, I had to reject thirteen members of a crew because they were too dehydrated to make the entry. They had all been partying the night before. I didn't know the crew leader at that point, but I had to keep walking up to him about every three minutes, saying, "So-

and-so flunked his test, so he can't make this entry. You've got to find another guy." I just kept going up, over and over, and rejecting members of his crew: "They can't go in. Sorry." And eventually that crew leader ended up becoming my husband. That's why I remember the year. But I didn't get a dinner invitation from him until after I bought Girl Scout cookies from his daughter. I remember thinking, *I'm on a remote island in the Pacific and somebody's selling Girl Scout cookies?* He sold four hundred boxes in two days. It was a taste of home we all had to have.

Johnston Atoll was also where I returned to formal education. After all those years of hauling bodies across highways and witnessing too many traumatic events, I realized that Dad was right. I should have a backup plan. As paramedics age and feel the toll that the job exacts on their bodies, they have to look for something else to do, and often they want to stick with a field they know. It's a natural progression. Health care still fascinated me, so I decided to become a nurse. There was a correspondence school on the island, and that was lucky for me. I earned my associate's degree in 1993 and transitioned to an RN right there.

In 1995, I moved to Casper, Wyoming, which is where my husband's parents lived, but then I got a job in Gillette, up in the northeast corner of the state. I initially started working for Hospice of Northeastern Wyoming as a hospice-care provider and then managed the organization for a year.

Hospice work is almost the opposite of emergency medical work. It's based on the idea of compassionate death: *how can we make end of life the most comfortable experience possible?* I really liked that work, because I got to go back into people's homes, create a caring environment, and prepare them to die as peacefully as they could. I stayed with hospice about fifteen months but, in rural Wyoming at that time, it came down to demographics. There weren't enough people who needed hospice, and I only got paid when I was actually caring for patients. So I went over to Custer, South Dakota, and took a full-time job as a staff medical-surgical nurse. Basically, I commuted about 125 miles once or twice a week, but I also found time to finish a bachelor's degree in 1998.

After my BSN, I thought I was pretty much done with my education, but late that same year, Excelsior College started a master of science in nursing program. They offered me a break on tuition if I'd be in their first cohort, and I said, "Okay, I'll try it out." You should understand that all of my education has been pay-as-you-go. I've never taken out student loans since my first year of college in 1979. I just work a lot and pay to go to school.

I finished in 2003 and thought, *Oh, good, I have a master's degree now. I'm all done with school. I shouldn't need anything else. I don't need a doctorate. I'm a working girl.* Famous last words. That was the start of a really expensive process – after two more master's degrees, I ended up going through the University of Massachusetts in Boston on their family nurse practitioner track. I wanted to be a nurse who could not only educate people about diabetes, but also have the ability to treat patients with the disease as well.

Currently, I work full time for an internal medicine clinic, Campbell County Clinics. As part of that, three mornings a week, I care for our nursing-home population. I'm also program director for our Diabetes Center. We do one-on-one education with each person, because we haven't found group classes to be effective. We ask relevant questions about their lifestyles: *What do you go through in a day? How do you manage? What aspect of diabetes do you want to work on first?* We let them set the path and help them find what works. Groups are great for support, for going to each other and saying, "I brought this new recipe. You should try it. It's really good." But when dealing with the nitty-gritty of the disease, I personally don't find groups specifically helpful.

I think the real answer is moderation. Normal blood sugars are normal blood sugars, and that's what we should try to achieve 80 percent of the time. For people with diabetes, we've got to cut them some slack. They're not perfect. They have a disease that's not ever going to allow their blood sugars to be perfect, so let's find a good place for them to be. Let's have them become knowledgeable and eat foods that the body was meant to have.

Diabetes is considered a personality problem. Our society tells you that it's your fault you have it. If you only ate right and exercised and did everything right, then you wouldn't have the disease. Even Type 1 people get branded with that mentality. What you have to remember is that 90 percent of the literature, as well as 90 percent of the people with diabetes, are Type 2. And even if you want to talk about the diabetics with Type 2, having the disease is still not necessarily their fault. There are eight known pathological defects in Type 2 diabetes, and those aren't defects that people volunteered to receive. You didn't tell your liver to over produce sugar. You didn't instruct your brain to ignore satiety signals. You didn't remind your guts to operate less effectively. And you certainly didn't send a signal to your pancreas to start dying off. Again, these are physiological defects, just as with Type 1 diabetes. But for some strange, punitive reason our society wants to link Type 2 diabetes with lifestyle choices. Regardless of that, diabetes is here to stay. It affects multitudes of people, and there is no one right way to treat it. It's about a lot of adaptations and about keeping people healthy. We can do anything with anybody who has diabetes, if we're creative enough to find an effective path, and I'm now dedicated to that endeavor.

You can live with diabetes and be healthy if you choose to get educated about it. Of everyone I've encountered with diabetes in a professional care environment, my guess would be that only 15 to 20 percent have enough passion and discipline about caring for themselves that they actually do what needs to be done. For a time, that was true with me, and it's true with my patients as well. I understand that it's a burden to check your blood sugar all the time, but that's just the beginning of what's necessary to stay healthy, and I'm thrilled that I can help. I have a broad opportunity as a nurse practitioner because I get to act as the primary care provider for my patients: I can identify their symptoms, educate them about the disease, help them manage it, and continually motivate them to have healthier lives

What I've learned again and again through all my different adventures is that you should never stop learning. If you're a professional, whatever your career path is – whether it's nursing or gardening or the professional being-at-home-mom track – there are always new things to learn. The world is constantly changing, and you have to be open to figuring out what else you should know. For me, of course, health care provides a professional sphere that is as rich and diverse as I could ever imagine. And even though I'm still a working girl, I did recently enter a doctoral program. Okay, I admit it, I'm addicted to school – mostly because I like to learn new things – but also because there's always an opportunity to figure out a better way to do what I try to do in health care.

IRINA VULAKH

*I grew up in Kiev, in the Ukraine, when
it was still part of the Soviet Union.
Because of my Jewish background, just
being accepted into nursing school was
an accomplishment, but I graduated and
worked as a nurse there twenty years ago.
I immigrated to New York City in 1997,
and studied on my own to become licensed
as a registered nurse in the United States.
Recently, I earned my MSN degree, which
allowed me to practice nursing at a higher
level in the emergency department at
the U.S. Naval Hospital Okinawa, which
is where my husband is stationed.*

My husband is active-duty military, so that's how I ended up in Okinawa. In the military hospital here, we train Navy corpsmen. They come out of the corpsman school, and this is their first chance to work in a hospital, so many of them don't really know what to do. The nurses have to teach them the basic skills, show them how to deal with patients, and train them for trauma cases. Doctors may assist with the training, but it is primarily the nurses' responsibility. We have to make sure we get them ready, because from here they may deploy to war zones like Afghanistan.

Primarily, I work in the emergency department, which is always busy. This is the largest overseas hospital for the United States military in the Pacific region. More than fifty thousand people on Okinawa alone are our beneficiaries, and we handle referrals for personnel and their families from islands and ships throughout the Pacific. I prefer working nights, usually the 6:00 p.m. to 6:00 a.m. shift, and I work because it makes me feel good. That may sound strange, but it's true. Right after I got married, my husband told me, "You don't have to work if you don't want to." But I work for me, and for my patients. It just makes me feel that I'm doing something with my life, that I'm helping people, and that I have a purpose.

Of course, there's always something going on at work that can get you upset, but for me it usually isn't the nursing part. Here in Okinawa, I only work part time, three or four days a week, and that makes the job easier. When I worked at the ER in Morgantown, West Virginia, I was on-call. If, for instance, there was a winter storm and people couldn't get to work, I lived five minutes from the hospital, and I could choose to work more than forty hours a week. But it wasn't something I had to do all the time.

I've seen nurses burn out because they worked so hard, especially in West Virginia, where the nurses I knew had families, and farms, and then they still carried full shifts every week. Often they were the only ones in their families who had jobs, so they couldn't just stop. They would get tired of not seeing their families, of commuting, of being there for so long, and tired of patients who kept coming in for simple problems. That happened way too often. It happens even here where our military patients don't have problems with insurance, but they still don't utilize the ER properly. They still come in for simple problems when they should be going to their primary-care doctors.

That doesn't bother me very much, though. If patients feel they have a reason to come into the ER, that's good enough for me. One of the doctors I like to work with says that what might look simple to us is still an emergency for the patient. I love being able to help with that emergency. We have admissions, of course, but most people go home the same day they come in. Sometimes they just need education. Here in Okinawa, for instance, we see lots of new parents. We do about a hundred deliveries a month, mostly with young parents who really need to know what to do with their babies. They're so grateful when somebody listens to them and explains what they should do. It's when they leave and say, "Thank you for helping me," that I remember again why I'm doing this.

Nursing is a hard job, especially emotionally. When I first went to nursing school, I don't think I realized how hard it would be. I was young. I thought, *I'm going to help people. I'm going to give them a drug for their pain and help them feel better.* Right after I finished eighth grade in Kiev, when I was fifteen, I entered a three-year nursing school. That was in 1988.

The Ukraine was still part of the Soviet Union at that time, and everything was controlled by the government. My family was Jewish, and that made everything harder for us. To get into nursing school, for example, you had to apply, and in Kiev most places would not take Jews.

It wasn't something they would state explicitly, but it was an unwritten rule. There was a line six on every application where they would ask your nationality and, if you wrote down Jewish, that was it. They would just pull your application out and not offer you the entrance exam. I believe my father had to go and bribe someone so I could get in.

After I graduated, I got a job at a center for eye surgery. It was one of the biggest eye centers in the Soviet Union. I thought I would be happy there. On my first day, they gave me a tour of the operating room during a surgery, saying things like, "This is what you're going to be doing. Your job is to assist the surgeons, pass instruments, or hold something when someone needs help." Now I had observed other kinds of surgeries when I was a nursing student, but I had never seen eye surgery before. Those other times, all the patients were unconscious. But this eye patient had crossed eyes, called strabismus, and they were operating to fix that condition, using a local anesthesia. He was completely conscious, although he couldn't feel any pain in his eye.

There are six muscles attached to each eye, and they control how the eyes move. One reason why people may have crossed eyes is because some of the muscles are weak and the other muscles have to compensate, and that eye may turn in or out, up or down. To repair the problem, they go in and change the shape or the position of the muscles to help the eyes line up the right way again. It's actually one of the bloodiest operations you can see in eye surgery, and it was the first one I had ever witnessed. Well, in the middle of the operation, the patient started talking to me. He could see me out of one eye, and he was saying I looked new – cute and fresh and green – something like that, smiling at me, and there was blood dripping out of the eye they were working on.

Suddenly, I felt nauseated. I had to leave the room. I found a corner and sank down. Then one of the anesthesiologists came out to check on me. I had turned white in the operating room, so he wanted to make sure I was all right. He was saying, "Everybody does that on their first day. It's going to be okay. You'll like it." And I was thinking, *Why am I here? Why was this my choice? Why did I decide to be a nurse? Is this really what I want to do every day of my life?* I was only eighteen years old at the time, and it was a really shocking experience. I went home after that. They gave me a day off to think about what had happened, and I went back in the next day, and it wasn't as bad the second time.

When I first started working with patients, I couldn't stop thinking about the job. At night, I even dreamed about it. I would wake up in the morning still tired because my brain had been processing images of the surgeries I had assisted on the day before – going back through, making sure everything I did was right for the patient and right for the doctor. Sometimes we had unsuccessful cases, not because the doctor had done something wrong but because we couldn't reverse a patient's blindness or some condition like that and, in my dream, I was still there, going through that, over and over, trying to make it successful.

I worked at the Center for Eye Surgery in Kiev for about six months before everything changed. I was actually at my job when they announced that there was no Soviet Union anymore. What usually happened when they had a problem in the government, or when one of the presidents died, was that they would have classical music playing on all the channels. Or they would put *Swan Lake* or some other ballet on. They wouldn't want people to panic so they didn't announce things right away. Of course, everyone knew something was wrong whenever that would happen, but none of us knew what was really happening.

It was scary. They flew Gorbachev somewhere, and they told us he was no longer president. They said that the Soviet Union didn't exist anymore – that the fifteen republics were separate countries – and right away there was some kind of war going on within Russia. A lot of police were in the streets, and that usually didn't happen. It was just very quiet. Nobody would smile or make a joke, because you didn't know who was listening. It was really unpleasant.

Once the Ukraine was separate, everything changed. The Center for Eye Surgery was privatized, and patients had to start paying for surgeries. We began to run out of supplies, and we would actually give our patients a list of supplies to bring with them if they wanted to have surgery. Eventually it got to the point that all of the resources were exhausted, and then the government had to step in. Then our pay went down almost fifty percent. We could see the bleak future that was coming, and everyone in my family began to leave the country.

In 1997 I moved to Brooklyn, where a lot of Russian people live. I was hired as a medical assistant for an American eye doctor in Brooklyn. Most of his patients were Russian, and he needed someone who understood eye diseases, was familiar with the terminology, and who also spoke their language. That's how I learned English. I didn't go to school for that. I learned it on the job.

When I was living in New York, I met my husband, who was in the Navy. Before I had a chance to study for my nursing license in America, he was transferred to Naples, Italy, where I passed my EMT boards and practiced emergency medicine for a year and a half. Once we were back in the United States, we moved to West Virginia, and that's where I passed my nursing boards and got my RN license. Since then, I've worked in hospital emergency rooms.

In West Virginia, I was surrounded by a group of very experienced nurses who taught me so much. When something tragic happened, they would tell me, "Don't let it get to you. Yes, it's sad. Yes, it's hard. But you can't let your next patients suffer. You can't let anything change the level of care you can provide for them."

I was very fortunate to work with people who shared their insights. Most of them worked the night shift. I asked them how they managed the job, and they said: "For some nurses, it becomes a routine. You will become exhausted, physically and emotionally, but you still have to find a way to sympathize with your patients without losing your perspective. Something difficult may happen in one room, but there are more patients in other rooms, and you have to be ready for them. It doesn't matter what problems they come in with – it could be a simple cold or it could be a heart attack. You have to continue to provide the same level of care, no matter what the problem is. Usually, you'll have to take care of something right away and then go back and try to explain to the people who are still sick, and are tired of waiting, that you're not trying to avoid them. You understand they've been waiting a long time. You understand they're sick, and they're upset. You can only get to them when you can, and when you do, you'll give each one the same high level of care. And at the end of the day, don't take the tragedies home with you, because you won't survive as a nurse."

That was good advice for me. Most of the time, I remember their words and try to follow them. Recently, though, it's been hard. We had a child die in our ER. He had pulled a heavy TV set off a table and sustained severe head trauma. The damage was so extensive that we couldn't save him. His mother was there, crying and screaming, and they were trying to contact her husband. That's one of the hardest times to be in the ER, when you can't do anything to comfort grieving parents. We have so much equipment and so many medications, but sometimes they can't help. I can usually dissociate myself and not carry the tragedies home, but this one really bothered me. I said to my husband, "Do you know what happened?" And he said, "Yes, but tell me about it." He knew I had to get it out. If every day at work were like that one, I probably wouldn't stay.

But most of my days are different. Most days, the work feels rewarding. People come in with pain and leave without pain. That's why I like the ER more than any other department. You can see the results of your efforts right away. When I see a person smile as they leave the ER, I know that we've accomplished something important. Most people don't get the chance to help anybody during their day. If I can help somebody go home feeling better, that small achievement makes it more than an ordinary day. I call that a wonderful day.

CLINT KNEUVEN

Currently I am a flight nurse with Memorial Hermann Lifeflight, which has been in business for thirty-five years. It was one of the first air medical providers in the country, and it serves an area within a 150-mile radius of Houston, Texas. I am licensed as a respiratory therapist, a paramedic, and a registered nurse.

Initially, when I was nineteen, I majored in business at a local community college. However, it didn't take me long to figure out I didn't care for economics. So I went to the counselor's office, and asked about the different degree programs they offered. In Houston, we have the Texas Medical Center, so the medical profession is a big employer in town. The counselor told me, "Hey, you can get a job pretty easy in health care." So I started going through their respiratory therapy program and I found out I liked it. That was in 1991, and I went on to work as an RT for fifteen years.

My day-to-day job as an RT depended on where I was working. If I was working in the hospitals, I was mainly taking care of ICU patients who were on ventilators, or had tracheotomies, or who were intubated. When I worked in the nurseries, I would respond to labor and delivery. I worked on a few high-risk preemie transports. Then when I worked in home care, it was kind of a completely different job. There, I was more going to people's houses and setting them up on oxygen equipment, or on C-PAP machines for sleep apnea.

When I was working as an RT at Herman, a 950-bed hospital here in the medical center, I stayed in the Level III nursery for ten of my fifteen years. They have an ECMO program there. ECMO stands for extracorporeal membrane oxygenation. Basically, it's a heart-lung bypass machine that takes the blood out of the body, oxygenates it, and then reintroduces it. On our ECMO team, there were nurses and RTs, and I was doing the same job the nurses were. I was administering blood and giving medicines through the pump, and I thought, *These nurses are doing the same thing I am and they're making a lot more money.*

I think I'll go to nursing school for this. So I enrolled, with the intention of remaining in the nursery at a higher salary.

One day, we had an infant on the ECMO pump. A perfusionist was sitting there watching, and he said, "Nobody can figure out what's going on with this thing. We can't get this kid off the bypass pump. So I said, "Let me see what I can do." And I realized pretty quickly the settings were off. Somebody had set it up wrong. "This pump's not running right," I said. "Look at it. You can tell it's going at the wrong speed."

"No," he said, "That's the right speed."

"It isn't. I'm telling you, it's the wrong speed."

So he calculated it and discovered it was out of calibration. "I can't believe you could tell by looking at it."

"Oh, yeah," I told him, "you sit here staring at this thing going around all day long and you can tell when it's not going at the right speed."

"Man, we've had fifteen people look at it, and you're the first one who figured it out."

Well, I didn't think much about it, but that interaction turned out to be important. Some of the perfusionists who worked on the machines with us also did transports of adult patients on balloon pumps, and that guy I had helped out was one of them. He asked if I wanted to try doing them, and I jumped at the chance. I began to do the transports, on a helicopter, shortly after I got out of nursing school.

I did them for a year, and then the director of the flight program said to me, "If you'd like to be a flight nurse, we're going to have an opening here in about nine months. Get your paramedic license, and we'd be interested in talking to you." So I went and enrolled in paramedic school after that and got my license.

I've been a flight nurse for about four years now, and it's probably the most interesting job you could have, period. From one day to the next, it's amazing. You see these shows on TV, and they try to sensationalize it, and even they can't make it out to be as cool as it really is. There are so many aspects to it. Basically, we do two different types of calls. One kind involves transports from one hospital to another. They'll call and say, "Hey, we've got somebody out here having a stroke." So we'll fly to this tiny community hospital that has absolutely no resources, and when we get there, we're it. We decide what needs to be done. We start them on whatever IV medicine they need. If they need to be intubated, we do that. We might put them on a ventilator. Then we load them onto a stretcher and fly them back to a larger hospital.

The other kinds of calls we do are called scene flights. Sometimes it will be a car accident, or a gunshot wound, or something like that, and they'll call us and say, "Hey, we need you to land on the freeway out here. We've got a three-car pileup." They'll shut the freeway down for us, and we'll land right in the middle of it to get those people out. Sometimes they might have an amputation or something like that, or hemorrhaging, those kinds of things. We'll do whatever interventions we need to do. We're the only flight service in the United States that carries blood and plasma on all of our flights with us, so we can administer either one en route to the hospital.

There's another paramedic who flies with me. I'm a nurse and a paramedic, and he's a flight paramedic. We're a two-man health care team. What we do is we trade out calls. One of us will go in the back of the ambulance while the other one prepares the stretcher. Then, on the following call, we'll switch roles. One time, we had this guy who was completely nuts. The cops told us, "Hey, be careful. We've got a guy who's high on PCP, and he tried to cut his throat." When we landed, it was the flight paramedic's turn to go in the back of the ambulance first.

So I was outside, standing near the back doors, and this cop said, "Yeah, we've been to this guy's house before. He's a drug addict." All of a sudden, the doors of the ambulance swung open, and there was this six-foot-tall guy, no clothes on, completely covered in blood. He was wrestling with the flight paramedic and also with the two EMTs. They were trying to get him onto the stretcher, and he was fighting all three of them. They had gloves on and they were trying to hold onto him, but he was naked and slippery from all the blood.

I could see where he had tried to cut his throat, but he had actually just about sawed his head off. He couldn't even hold it up, because he had cut so many of the muscles in his neck. His head was kind of bobbing back and forth, and every time it would bob back, his windpipe would poke out like a turkey neck. It was surreal. The flight paramedic looked down at me and said, "I could use your help in here." I said, "Okay, I'll be right there," and I jumped up into the back.

They didn't have an IV on this guy to sedate him. They were just holding him down. We have this tool that lets you drill into somebody's shinbone and establish rapid access for an IV. He was still struggling like crazy, so I held his leg down and drilled it into his shin. Then I pulled out some meds to sedate him. I looked at them and said, "Now I'm going to paralyze him. Are you going to be able to get an ET tube in his airway?" My partner looked at me and said, "Yeah, I think so. I'm holding his trachea in my hand."

So I pushed in the meds and paralyzed the guy, and the flight paramedic stuffed the ET tube into this guy's trachea that was hanging out. Blood was everywhere, and I figured he must have bled out most of his volume. Anyway, we tied him down to the stretcher real quick. He was still leaking all over the place, and we lost his heartbeat. We were doing chest compressions and trying to stop the bleeding at the same time. By the time we landed, he had bled so much they couldn't save him. That PCP, it's a drug that won't stop. The cops told us, "Yeah, you get these guys who are high on PCP and you shoot them and they just keep coming at you."

I don't usually get freaked out by the bloodier calls. Some people do. But I also don't like to use the expression, "used to it." You don't want to get so calloused that you become used to terrible events. You need to stay focused. It's one of those things where, when you're in the middle of it, you start thinking, *Okay, what do I need to do now? And what do I need to do next?* If I sit and feel awful about what's going on at the time, I'm already behind the eight ball. I've got to get in front of it. That's kind of the secret to it: you've got to be thinking five steps ahead of where you're at now, so you don't get yourself painted into a corner with something. You really don't have a whole lot of time to let compassion cloud your judgment.

I remember one time they called us out for a seventeen-year-old kid who had decided he was going to ride his dirt bike out in this open field.

He was zipping across the field at some high rate of speed, and he was in shorts and tennis shoes – no shirt, no helmet, no protective gear on at all. And while he was speeding along, he hit a ditch, and it threw him off the bike. He face-planted into a telephone pole, and the skin just about peeled off. In the back of the ambulance, I remember seeing his face all swollen up and the paramedics pumping air into him with the mask because he wasn't able to breathe on his own. But they needed to put an ET tube into him, too, and they were having a difficult time doing that.

One of the key things we do is to help people manage their breathing. So I was looking at this kid, and each time they pressed, the air would actually squirt out of his scalp. The impact had de-gloved the skin from his face and scalp, and one of the paramedics actually had to go and throw up outside the door. That's part of it, too. In the middle of these things, you've got to really try to hold it together emotionally and psychologically, but sometimes your body just betrays you physiologically.

No matter what happens, you've got to hang in there and get the job done. You can't say it out loud, but you're going through your list, thinking, *Okay, I know this looks crazy, but the first thing we need to do is get this guy secured. Let's get an IV in him. Let's get an airway in him. Let's get the airway secured. Let's get him on a stretcher.* That's the organized way that you have to be thinking the whole time that your patient is looking all messed up and just trying to survive the trauma.

Some people get off on the gore, where somebody has lost a leg or something terrible like that. But often those can be easier cases. For instance, with a car accident, you can go in there and put a tourniquet on to stop the bleeding, and then you make sure their airway is controlled. You give them some sort of volume, probably blood in this case, and you rush them to where they can do a surgical intervention. So it's usually those three first: stop the bleeding, control the airway, and provide volume. It often looks gory, but it's actually easier. You've got to move quickly, though. It's a fast-paced thing. If you pull somebody out of the back of a car and they're bleeding out, you've got to prioritize what needs to be done immediately.

I remember this one call that set up a real dilemma for me. We got a call out to this local hospital, probably about five minutes away. So we flew out there and went into the ER, and there was this six-month-old kid who was on this warmer in the ER. There must have been fifty people running around in this room. I tried to get a report: "What's going on? What happened here?"

They told me the baby's mom was at home and the father had barged in and taken the six-month-old kid hostage. He had locked himself in the bedroom and taken a box cutter to him. This poor kid had stab wounds all over his abdomen and chest. Somehow the mom had finally gotten the kid away from the dad and taken him to an ER. That's where we picked him up and flew him to a trauma center.

When we got back to the base and were sitting in the break room, the TV was on and the story was on the news. The dad was still locked inside the apartment and, as we were watching it live, the SWAT team crashed in there. All of a sudden, you could hear the actual gunshots. I just grabbed my radio and said, "We're fixing to get a call." And within two minutes, sure enough, they called us.

Of course, we had to fly out there and pick up the dad. He had tried to cut his own throat with the same box knife. I had to take care of this guy who, an hour before, had sliced up his infant son. For a second, part of me wanted to let the guy die, to exact some kind of crude justice, but I couldn't act on that. My job is not to be the judge and jury of what somebody does. I have to treat everybody the same, whether it's a drunk driver who ran into a car and killed four people or it's the kid who was in the back of a car without a seat belt on. My job isn't to decide – that's God's job.

There was another guy, I remember, who was having a heart attack. It was kind of funny, speaking of God's job. We flew to this hospital that's out in this very rural part of Texas. It looked like a little nursing home out in the country, and they had a small concrete helipad next to it. We had to pick up this guy who was probably in his fifties. I bundled him up and was walking next to him as we got back out to the helipad. He said, "You see this helipad you guys landed on? My dad built this when I was a kid."

I looked at him and said, "If nothing else has come full circle in your life, this moment right here has." Think about the coincidence: when this guy was a kid, his father was a concrete contractor who built a helipad in front of a hospital in the middle of nowhere. And now, fifty years later, we could land on that helipad, pick him up when he was having a heart attack, and fly him to a hospital that would save his life. What's that line about God working in mysterious ways?

I think back on the nineteen-year-old kid that I was, and I remember I was just looking for a curriculum where I wouldn't have to take economics. My whole career has actually been a series of little things that, at the time, didn't seem like a big deal, but which ended up completely changing my direction. Like the day I found the ECMO pump that was spinning at the wrong speed – if I hadn't found that, who knows what would have happened?

There's a strange story that illustrates how chance has operated in my life. Every time I think about this, I feel like I'm meant to be doing what I'm doing. When the program director of the flight program said to me, "Hey, if you want to be a flight nurse, we'll be interested in talking to you, but you need to get your paramedic license," I was thirty-five and had just gone through a divorce. My ex-wife had split and left me to raise our eleven-year-old son, and right then I had this guy ask me if I wanted to do this whole new thing. I was thinking, *You've got to be kidding me*, but I just said, "Yeah, okay."

So I went down to the college and applied to get my paramedic training. They told me, "We'll do this accelerated program for you, since you're already a nurse. That way, it won't take as long. You could probably knock it out in a couple of semesters. Go ahead and enroll in these two classes here, and then later on in the semester, we'll let you know the other classes you'll have to take."

So I was sitting there, totally broke, and trying to figure out how I could do everything. I was working full time as a nurse during the day, taking night classes to earn my paramedic license, and trying to raise my son as a single father, all at the same time. And I was thinking, *God, I don't know what's coming up next semester. If they hit me with some full-time schedule, I'm not going to be able to do this. I can't even afford books right now.* I was trying to go through paramedic school, basically, with no books.

My advisor was one of the instructors in my program. One night, I finished my last class, and it was probably 9:30. I was taking these classes way on the other side of town, and I still had to drive home. It was about an hour's drive. Well, I had almost gotten out to my car and I said to myself, *I've got to go talk to this guy. I can't keep doing this, working until 7:00 at night, going to school until 9:30, driving home, picking my kid up from the sitter, then falling in bed so I can get up at 5 a.m. and go to work the next day. Doing all this is just wearing me out. I don't know if I can complete this paramedic program. I'm broke, and this is crazy. Why am I doing this?*

I walked back to the classrooms in the school, and all the lights were out. I walked down this dark hallway, and the only light that was still on was in my advisor's office. *Good, he's still there.* But when I reached his office, he wasn't in there. However, just inside there was this empty desk, and the two paramedic books I couldn't afford to buy were sitting on top of it. There was a hand-lettered sign tacked above them that said, *FREE: Take these.* So I took them, and I never looked back.

The absolute best part of my job is when my patients go home after experiences that almost killed them. People go through their lives and, for the most part, they raise a family and go to work and just try to enjoy those lives. Then something happens – a car wreck, a stroke, an accident, a heart attack, or some other traumatic event. In the hour after that, they live or they die. When I can help them live, the feeling is impossible to describe. There are even days where I get to save two or three lives. Sometimes I'll go and see my patients in the hospital the day after, and they're so grateful for what I did that they'll start to cry. Nothing can compare to that feeling.

MARGARET CHANDLER

I graduated with my associate's degree in fall 2004, and with my bachelor's degree in 2007. Since then, I have worked in emergency and critical-care areas, as well as in ground-based specialty care transport. I have maintained board certifications as a CEN, CCRN, CTRN, and CFRN. My BSN allowed me to commission into the Air Force Reserve as a nurse in 2008. Currently, I'm pursuing a master's degree to achieve licensure as an acute-care nurse practitioner.

The day I decided to go to nursing school, I was working as a paramedic in Jersey City, New Jersey. My unit assignment for the day was the specialty-care transport unit, the SCTU, a specially equipped ambulance dispatched not just to homes or accident scenes but also to hospitals to transfer patients whose care requirements were too complex for the sending facility to manage.

Bob, the nurse I was working with that day, was very sharp. Nothing seemed to rattle him, whether it was a desperately ill ICU patient on a dizzying array of IV drips or the 911 dispatch for a baby who wasn't breathing. He also pulled his weight when it was time to do the tedious and often dirty work involved in keeping an ambulance in service and ready for the next call. Bob had worked as a paramedic before he went to nursing school, and he understood how to be a good partner.

It was no secret in the department that the nurses got paid far better than the paramedics did. Bob always picked up the tab for his crew when we got coffee. I was newly certified, broke, and working two jobs, regularly pulling five or six twelve-hour shifts a week, so I appreciated Bob's gesture. We had just completed a transfer and were drinking coffee in the parking lot when he asked me, "So when are you going to nursing school?"

It might sound like a small thing, but I wanted to be able to afford coffee for the crew the way Bob could, and I also wanted to be able to do more for my patients. I loved working as a paramedic, and I still do, but I knew that my options for advancement in EMS were limited. I knew, from looking at some of my coworkers, that all of my overtime would catch up with me eventually. And after six years on the SCTU, full of long periods of boredom interrupted by moments of sheer terror, as they say, I also knew that ninety-nine out of every hundred runs struck me as more boring than terrifying.

That isn't to say I didn't find joy in my job. It gave me a different perspective on patients, because for the first time, I had time to really talk to people. Sometimes, when people are going in for a procedure in a catheterization lab, for instance, they get downright philosophical, especially when you tell them they may wind up needing heart surgery. I saw and heard some amazing things. I remember, in Newark, there was an elderly African American woman who looked pretty frail. She had alopecia from having her hair in braids for most of her life. I couldn't tell much about her by simple observation. When we got her settled in, she looked at me and said, "You know, the only thing I really regret in my life is that I didn't go for that doctoral degree."

I remember a hypoglycemic in Bayonne who was trying to kill us all. It was about 3:00 a.m. and there was this little crucifix on the wall. Somebody hung the IV bag on that because there was no other place to put it, and the patient was going wild. He grabbed the IV tube and yanked it out of the bag and stood there, laughing at us. It was downright cinematic. When we finally wrestled him down and got some D50 into him, he became the sweetest person alive. He just wanted to bake us cookies.

I remember a kid who was running for a bus in Jersey City and was so focused on catching the bus that he ran straight into a light pole. He was screaming and freaking out at first, and I was on the radio, trying to calm him down and telling the doc I wanted to administer some morphine. And the kid yelled, "Morphine? Oh, not morphine." Then I gave it to him, and he stared up at me from the stretcher and said, "Sweetie, I like you."

A lot of that time blurs together now because I took care of so many different kinds of people. In Jersey City, we treated folks all along the economic spectrum, from absolute destitution to outrageous wealth, and guess what I learned: everybody gets sick and, at some point, everybody needs help.

---------------------------- * ----------------------------

Early on, my parents instilled the importance of service in me. They were both volunteers, and at Christmas we always went to the fire department in Ironia, New Jersey, and put together packages for local kids who wouldn't get Christmas presents any other way. I think I got my sense of duty from that. At home, their beepers would go off, and they'd jump up, get dressed really fast, and take off to go help somebody. For a four-year-old, that passed for glamour and excitement, as if they were hurrying into a phone booth and then emerging in tights and a cape. It left a huge impression on me.

When I was nine, we moved, and my parents split up shortly after that. After I entered high school, all the volunteer stuff went away. I went off to college at the University of Delaware, and I graduated with two majors, political science and geography, a full year early. I was determined to save the world. I was going to become an environmental lawyer and prosecute environmental racism cases. If you had told me as an eighteen-year-old undergraduate that I was going to wind up working in health care, I think I would have been horrified.

After graduation, I moved in with my dad and stepmother so I could live on the cheap and pay off college debts. I took the LSATs, planned to enter law school, and scored an entry-level job in government relations. But I was feeling isolated, so every Friday night, I'd drive from North Jersey to Newark and hang out with college friends. On my way back from one particularly boring Labor Day weekend there, I just got this sudden flash: *I want to join a rescue squad.* I was twenty-one, my parents were divorced, and I felt aimless. It wouldn't take more than a freshman survey class in psychology to help someone conclude that the idea of rescuing people in distress might have appealed to me around that time. And that's when I fell down the rabbit hole.

In 1997, I started volunteering in Central Jersey. I was paying my bills with office work, but all I wanted to do was get home and jump on the ambulance. So I enrolled in paramedic school and interviewed for an EMT job in East Orange, which is kind of like Newark, only smaller, and there's no legal economy there. I walked in carrying a briefcase, and a man named Dave Strange, the medic on duty said, "Sorry, the social worker's office is downstairs."

"No, I'm here for the EMT interview," I said. "I just got admitted to medic school, and I need to know what a bad night on the ambulance is like."

"Okay, you're hired," he said.

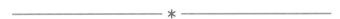

Four years after that, I was still a rookie paramedic and working in Jersey City on September 11, 2001, when we became the triage point for the thousands of people fleeing from Manhattan in ferries across the river. We had a flood of refugees, but we also had to deal with every volunteer fire department, or rescue squad, or community watch that showed up in Jersey City and said, "Hey, we're here to help." Their hearts were definitely in the right place, but we were overwhelmed just trying to find places for these people to park their ambulances and go to the bathroom. They all wanted to go dig people out of the pile, but they didn't have any sense of chain of command. In the meantime, if you needed an ambulance in Caldwell or Piscataway or Dumont, you were probably out of luck.

Eventually, we did go into Manhattan that night. The intel was sketchy but we had reports that there were a lot of people who needed help at a makeshift hospital in Battery Park City. Initially, our director didn't want to be short-staffed and didn't want to lose any of us. Finally, she relented. We wanted to help, of course, but we also felt the volunteer folks wouldn't survive in that environment. Nobody's radio worked well because the communication towers were down, and if somebody had gotten lost or hurt, it would have taken a long time to track them down. The volunteer companies weren't thinking of it that way because they didn't have any mass-casualty training. Some of them went over, but it was under our watch.

It was nightmarish, it was absurd, and it was poignant. There really wasn't a whole lot going on at that point. We went to Battery Park, and we irrigated a lot of eyes. We mobilized people to get them over the river and back safely. We didn't lose anybody who was working with us that day. But one of our report chiefs worked for Port Authority, and he was one of the thirty-seven guys who didn't make it out. He'd been told not to run in, but he did. "No, really, you have to let me go," was the last thing he said.

The morning after, we were walking through Battery Park and the toxic dust was everywhere. It looked like it was snowing. It looked like nuclear fallout in one of the *Terminator* movies. We walked by a guy asleep on a bench under some newspapers, and one of the girls from the volunteer squad cried out, "Oh, my God, there's a dead body over there." Somebody consoled her, but the medic with me resorted to the gallows humor that we use to survive tragic events and said, "Are you kidding? That SOB is the first guy in lower Manhattan to get back to his regular routine. God bless him." That weak joke didn't help us for long, though. There was the sense that nothing was ever going to be the same again. The truly horrifying part of it was that the dead bodies were floating in the air around us and we were breathing them in.

All we did was work for days. It was a way to keep our minds from dwelling on the tragedy. And while I worked, I had the realization that 9/11 wasn't going to be a one-time event. We were facing a future of mass casualty incidents, and I really wanted to learn the best ways to manage them. I felt that if I went into the military, I could get that organizational knowledge, but I wanted to go in as a nurse. So I enrolled in nursing school, earned my associate's degree in 2004 and my bachelor's in 2007. That BSN allowed me to commission into the Air Force Reserve in 2008. I am currently a captain serving in the 514th Aerospace Medicine Squadron at Joint Base McGuire-Dix-Lakehurst, New Jersey, where I train airmen to be instructors in SABC, the Air Force combat lifesaving class.

---- * ----

Since my licensure as an RN, I have worked in the emergency department, the cardiothoracic ICU, and the critical-care float pool, but I've never stopped working as a paramedic. I definitely identified more as a paramedic for the first few years that I had my nursing license. I'd be driving to work at the ICU, wishing and praying for an accident so I wouldn't have to go in and work on the ward with the other nurses.

To be a good nurse, to have a love for this profession and work at the beside, it involves a lot of tilting at windmills. I think it's impossible to do it the way we feel it ought to be done in the circumstances where we find ourselves. The profession can break your heart, literally and figuratively, and defense mechanisms differ. Some nurses wear themselves out attempting to conform to a standard of perfection and don't have any tolerance for someone who doesn't also martyr herself. I'll be the first to throw my gender under the bus: I think that's an especially feminine approach, and I think it drives a lot of the lateral violence.

The whole "nurses eat their young" concept isn't anything new. My take on it is that nurses engage in lateral violence because the people who are the most intimidated by the potential of nursing are nurses. Whenever I've seen an older nurse take a newer nurse down a peg, I've thought that the underlying message behind that is, *I'm only allowed to do so much. How dare you have the temerity to act as if you're smarter than that, or you're more valuable than that?* Part of that is pecking order, but it's also the idea that if someone has low self-esteem and is territorial, and then a new person who is idealistic and enthusiastic and fresh-faced shows up, that's going to chafe.

Now there are older, experienced nurses who are tremendous advocates for new nurses, and there are younger nurses who engage in lateral violence themselves. But sometimes I think that if someone has already traded some of her autonomy in for not having responsibility, it's a little galling to see somebody new who hasn't made that same decision.

Some people just get cynical, some go away, and others say, "Okay, well, I can't get all the starfish back into the ocean, but I can get this one in." However, while you're out there on the beach throwing starfish back into the ocean, you have to do a little bit of risk management for yourself. When you find yourself thinking, *I know that the best thing for this 270-pound post-op patient is to get him up out of bed and into a chair,* you had best remember that you weigh 130 pounds, have only one nursing aide, and there are eighteen more patients on your floor. Go find some help.

As professionals and nurses, we enjoy safeguards that exist today because the nurses who went before us rattled cages and said, "No, I'm not going to work without gloves. No, I'm not going to work with mandatory overtime. No, I'm not going to let the surgeon throw equipment around just because he's got a temper." So what are the answers to the problems that persist? Part of the answer is that we have to be vigilant about managing physical and professional risks. But we also have to manage emotional risks. How much will we allow ourselves to feel?

Coming from an EMS background, this is an issue that I've really struggled with. Nobody holds physicians accountable for what's going on in their interior emotional landscapes the way we do with nurses, and I still haven't quite figured out what my stance is on that. When I was doing my BSN, professors talked about the idea of professional caring and emotional response. My initial reaction to that was, "If I'm providing competent treatment to my patients, what difference does it make how I feel about it?"

Part of it has to do with my attention span. I like finding the problem, fixing it, and moving on. I love talking to people. I like getting intensively involved in a problem for an hour. I'll sit there and talk to you while they're cutting you out of your car. I'll sit there and comfort your family as you're being resuscitated. I'll even deal with the discussions that spook some nurses, like death notifications with families. Not a problem for me.

But I burn out far faster when I have to deal with the same patient for multiple days in a row. I don't know why. Maybe I can only be authentically present like that when I know it's time-limited. It may just be my comfort zone from growing up in EMS first. Maybe a logical approach makes more sense to me. I like coming in, solving the problem, and moving on. Being task-oriented probably protects me emotionally, and makes it a whole lot easier to truly hang it up at the end of a shift.

Here's the way I feel: *I didn't give you the heart attack; I didn't steer your car into the train; I didn't overdose your baby on the cough medicine. I'm not responsible for what happened to you, but I will show up and I will do the job to the best of my ability*. Patients don't want somebody who looks as if they're out of control. They want someone who's capable. They want someone who shows up looking pressed out and squared away. What bothers me most is when I feel as if I wasn't able to do what I was supposed to do because of low staffing, because of inadequate resources, or because I didn't know any better.

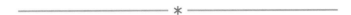

These days, I work in the ER at Hackensack, and a pay period doesn't go by when I'm not interpreting EMS to nursing and nursing to EMS. I definitely look at things like a paramedic sometimes, even when I'm acting as a nurse. It's situationally based: which discipline serves the patient better at a particular moment? They're different philosophies, with different preparations and, to be honest, EMS is a better preparation for certain circumstances. If you're injured, you want paramedics there to get you through the first forty-five minutes. We're outward, and we're goal-driven. But paramedics are trained to think about it differently – the goal is patient survival. It's a technical preparation as opposed to a professional one, and I don't believe that EMS is a profession. Emergency medicine can't really ever truly lay claim to its own body of work: it borrows from medicine, from nursing, and from public safety. Nursing, however, does have its own body of knowledge. There are things that nursing has an expertise in that nobody else does.

Nursing is an excellent profession, and it's a great way to thrive and survive in the health care industry. There are a lot of people who work in emergency medicine who feel the way I did: they want to stay in health care, but they need to make a better living. It's often the difference between, "I can respond first, take care of sick people, work seventy-hour weeks, and never be able to afford a mortgage," or, "I can do it this other way and have a better chance of surviving my career and not breaking my back." One of the major problems with EMS is that the ladder is pretty short: you can become the boss or you can become the educator, and that's about it for long-term options. In that respect, nursing is much better. It's a big tent, and it shelters a lot of different types.

I've been a nurse for eight years now – not very long in the grand scheme of things – but I've already gotten to work in the emergency department and in specialty ICUs. And I get to travel to places like Mozambique on nursing missions or to Gulfport, Mississippi, as a subject-matter expert, helping the Air Force improve its operational readiness for MCIs.

There aren't many professions that will offer you that range of experience or present so many options for new responsibilities.

I'm studying to be a nurse practitioner now because I like the idea of providing primary care to patients, but I also like the idea that I could be a resource for nurses who deliver essential bedside care. Not to rely on an old cliché, but you can give someone a fish, and they'll have one meal, or you can teach someone how to fish, and they'll be able to feed themselves forever. I'll take the long-term option any day of the week.

FRANCESCA LIND

I grew up in Frankfurt, Germany, and in Vicenza, about thirty miles north of Venice, speaking Italian, German, and English. I came to the United States in 1998 with my husband, and we lived on Whidbey Island, near Seattle. I learned about an LPN program at Skagit Community College in Oak Harbor, and that's where my nursing career started. I finished my BSN in December 2011, and I am currently studying to be a nurse practitioner in mental health.

I was living in Vicenza the summer I met my husband, working in the kitchen at the military base there, and he was my boss. Seven months later we were married, and seven months after that, he retired. We moved to Coupeville, on Whidbey Island, in the Puget Sound, and sunshine went out of my life. Don't get me wrong: it's a beautiful place, but I'm a sun person, and three-quarters of the time, it's raining or overcast there. I had to visit a tanning salon to help with seasonal disorder.

I worked at a K-mart, where I met this young Filipino lady who used to come in all the time. One day I said, "What do you do?" She said, "I'm going to nursing school," and she told me about the community college in Oak Harbor. I told my husband I wanted to become a nurse, and he said, "Go for it." So I enrolled in September, and I was an LPN one year later, in 2002. I got a job almost immediately in a nursing home.

While I was working there, I found an online school where I could study on my own and do the clinical at my own facility because it was skilled nursing. I called an official at the Washington State Board of Nursing who said, "Yes, as long as you have a nurse with a master's degree, and she signs off on your internship, you need four hundred hours of clinical there before you can take the state board exam." So by the time I finished all the classes, I had also done my four hundred hours. I drove to Spokane, took my state boards, and was licensed as a registered nurse in 2005.

As soon as I became an RN, I found a second job off the island in Everett, Washington, on a medical-surgical floor in the hospital there. The new nurses I worked with told me to get out of the nursing home, but I didn't want to leave. I enjoyed it there and, in some ways, it even felt like my home. "You're going to have a hard time getting a job in a good hospital. A lot of people don't think RNs who work in nursing home are competent nurses. You lose your skills in a nursing home," they told me. Maybe I shouldn't have listened to them. I went and worked full time in Everett on the med-surg floor and, within eight months I was divorced.

I decided to move to Corpus Christi, Texas. My stepdaughter was there for her first year in college, and I wanted to be near her. But Spohn Hospital, which is one of the biggest hospitals in Corpus Christi, also offered me a year's contract, with a $10,000 signing bonus, so that made it a little easier. I worked in their urology unit, and I also found another job at Corpus Christi Heart Medical Center, and I started in their telemetry unit so I could move to an ICU later on.

Near the end of 2007, I became a travel nurse. I was hired by a private agency to go and work in different hospitals. Sometimes I would have a three-month contract, sometimes six months. Once, I stayed for nine months in North Carolina because I really liked the hospital there. I was going between North Carolina, Texas, and Arizona. There was a nursing shortage, and the money was great. At certain jobs, I was making $75 an hour. The agency paid for my apartment and all my utilities. The only things I had to cover were my cell phone and the gas for my car. And on my days off, I could drive around and see new parts of the country.

My last contract ended in January 2009. It was supposed to go until March of that year, but the economy had soured. A friend I had known for thirty years lived in Colorado Springs, so I decided to move there. But when I arrived, the economy wasn't any better. All the hospitals had hiring freezes in place. I contacted a local nursing agency, and the only job available was for an infirmary nurse in the El Paso County Jail, so I took it.

I was in the main infirmary, and I had to answer every code. Any time somebody was coding, there was a rapid response, and I had to go with deputies to an area where there could be a hundred inmates, free and roaming around. That was scary. But I learned that if you respect them, they usually leave you alone. But I also found out that inmates know how to lie through their teeth to get any type of medicine you will give them, even if they don't need it.

I had this inmate who faked a seizure so well I thought it was real until I said, "Let me get some Ativan from my bag." Ativan helps to relax muscles and stabilize breathing so people don't suffer post-seizure problems. All of a sudden he woke up and said, "Oh, no, you can't give me Ativan. I'm allergic to it." That inmate knew he had court the next day where he would be given a life sentence with no parole. So maybe he thought he could postpone his court date.

One night, though, I really did get scared. We had a bad storm, and I was in the infirmary with three patients who were there for mental health issues. They were green-vest patients. A green vest means they're completely naked, except for this green vest that looks like a double apron. Velcro strips hold it together on the sides. Green-vest patients had to stay in cells with thick doors and three electric locks, and they have no bedding. They have a very small mattress, and they get finger foods because they're on suicide watch. If they want to kill themselves, almost anything can become a weapon. They have to stay down in the infirmary, away from everybody else, until they get evaluated by mental health.

Well, that one storm was so bad the electricity went out. The infirmary turned completely black for about ten seconds before the generator kicked in. Those ten seconds felt like an hour. I stood there, thinking, *They're going to pull those doors open and assault me. I'm by myself in here*. I had a walkie-talkie but, in the dark, you can't see which button is the alarm button. So I said a prayer, "God, please, make sure I'll be okay," and ten seconds later the generator started, and the lights came on. I jumped then, because the lieutenant was standing next to me. It was so black inside there I didn't see him come in.

I couldn't stay in that job. It got worse and worse. We had illegal immigrants coming through all the time, and they posed a terrible health risk. Immigration and Customs Enforcement would bring in about a hundred immigrants at a time, and we'd have to check them in and examine them. They carried all sorts of contagious problems – crab lice, weird skin disorders, strep throat, pinkeye. We had to quarantine them until they recovered, and we were always concerned we would have an epidemic in the jail. All the inmates used the same bathrooms and showers, and they could catch something pretty easily.

After about six months at the jail, I got a job in the military hospital at Fort Carson. I worked in the ICU for a year, and then I moved down to the emergency department. I love the ER. I feel like this is what I was meant to do. I must have ADHD, because I can never stay still. I need to stay busy, and this ER definitely keeps me busy.

Fort Carson is strictly a military hospital. We only serve military families. I hate to admit this, but I have seen a lot more abuse here than at other places I've worked. I work night shifts with this one doctor and, whenever we work together, we always get abuse cases. I told him, "I'm going to change my schedule."

One of the worst cases of starvation abuse was exactly three weeks ago. I had this baby who was eight months old and weighed only about six pounds. Have you ever seen an alien baby? Have you ever watched those movies where they show you this little green alien? They've got this big old head, but the baby's bald and very small. You can almost see their bones. That's what we call "an alien baby" in the hospital.

So this baby looked like that. His mom told us the child was a "failure to thrive" baby. The baby didn't want to eat, didn't want to drink, didn't want to be nurtured. Every time she tried to feed him, he vomited. I said, "Well, okay. It could be the gastric flu." It was me and this particular doctor again, and when I saw the baby, the first thing I said to him was, "Doctor, this isn't failure to thrive. I think it's another abuse case."

The mother was a military wife, and the father was deployed somewhere overseas.

When I took the baby's clothes off, I got that anger moment. I wanted to start yelling, "How can you do this to your own child?" But I had to stay objective, so I asked about the child's history: vaginal delivery, nine pounds at birth, fifty centimeters long, no complications.

Nine pounds at birth, and eight months later he had dropped to six pounds?

"What did you do when you noticed that your child lost all that weight in such a short amount of time?" I said. "Did you take him to your pediatrician for a well-baby check?" And the mother said the weirdest thing to me: "I didn't know how to set up a doctor's appointment." Then, a few minutes later when the doctor came into the room, she said, "I scheduled a follow-up appointment the first time I noticed he lost weight," and she gave us her pediatrician's name. We couldn't find the pediatrician she named anywhere in Colorado. Worse than that, she hadn't come to our military facility to have her baby. She went to an outside hospital, and she never reported on post that the baby had been born. There was no paperwork stating that she was even pregnant, so she hadn't come for prenatal care, either.

The baby was dehydrated, and I said to the doctor, "We've been working together for quite a while, and you know I'm good at what I do. If you trust me as a nurse, let me take some Pedialyte and try to feed this baby." Pedialyte is almost like Gatorade, but for children. There's no milk. You give it to children if they've got an upset stomach or they're vomiting, and it helps to restore fluids with all the electrolytes that they need. I said "If it's really failure to thrive, then the baby won't want to drink or even try to suck on the nipple of the baby bottle." He said, "You're right. I hadn't even thought about that."

I went and got a Pedialyte, but because he had been so malnourished, I couldn't feed him too much at once. I tried with two ounces, and the baby stuck his mouth on that baby bottle like there was no tomorrow. And I said, "This is not failure to thrive. This is failure to feed on the mom's part." By the time we transferred him, he had drunk sixteen ounces of Pedialyte, and he never vomited, never had diarrhea, and he started to become more alert. I said, "This baby has to be taken away from the mom."

So we called Child Protective Services, and we had to call the MPs, the military police, and the Colorado Springs Police. If you're a nurse or a doctor, it's mandatory to report child abuse. We can't follow up on the cases because that would violate the HIPAA laws, but sometimes we'll hear news reports about what happens.

I usually don't take problems from work home with me, but that starvation baby affected me so much that I couldn't sleep. Every time I closed my eyes, I saw that alien baby's crying face. When I went into work the next day, I talked to my charge officer, and he said, "Yeah, I know your case. If you want, I'll call the hospital to see how he's doing." When he called, the nurse there told him, "He's eating like a pig. Don't worry. Everything is good. We'll fatten him up." Once I heard that, I relaxed. I had no problems sleeping the next morning after my shift.

That one was personal. I have one child who will turn twenty next month. He was a miracle child, because I was supposed to be infertile. After he was born, I tried to have another, but doctors told me I couldn't have more children, and that turned out to be true. Seeing someone treat a baby like that made me furious. That baby's mother starved him on purpose? Where is God sometimes?

In my LPN class, we started with forty-five students. Only fifteen graduated. Out of that fifteen, only five still work as nurses. Everybody else quit. They burned out, or they gave up searching for jobs, or changed careers. What a waste. Maybe people burn out because they let all these different cases, like starving babies, take away their strength and their purpose.

I love nursing. I love taking care of people and feeling useful to others. And love to learn from others, even my own patients. Whenever someone tells me, "I'd like to go to nursing school," I tell them, "This is hard, rewarding work, but don't let the bad parts get to you. Find a way to stay fulfilled."

CYNTHIA SMATHERS

I started out many years ago wanting to be a nurse, but then I found respiratory therapy. I worked as an RT for over thirty-five years, including twenty-eight of them as a program director for a large private school, and I raised my son as a single mother. I had obtained my master's in education and counseling for my job, but I couldn't pursue my nursing dream until much later in my life. I graduated in 2005, obtained my RN license in February 2006, and now work for Hospice of the Valley, the largest, oldest, and only nonprofit hospice provider in Arizona.

There is one patient I'll always remember. He came to hospice on a Friday afternoon, so he had not yet been assigned a case manager or social worker. But his pain symptoms were out of control, and my team of continuous care nurses went in for the weekend to see if we could help manage them. He was relatively young – fifty years old – and married, with a wife who was probably twenty years younger, and two children, seven and nine. He had rectal cancer, and his tumors had extruded through his groin. It was horrific. That brave man, he wanted to take as little pain medication as possible. He wanted to teach his children whatever he could in the time he had left, and he needed to stay alert to talk with them.

Unfortunately, because of the tumors, he was completely bent over. His chest was almost touching his knees, and he was forced to lean to one side in his chair. When I came in, I said, "Would you be more comfortable in bed?" And he said, "I haven't straightened up in three months. Don't touch me. Don't go anywhere near that area. There's just too much pain." You could tell with one look he was a fighter, but there was no way to fight what he had.

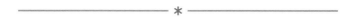

I was already in my early fifties when I became a nurse. When I was younger, I had been torn between going to nursing school and becoming trained in respiratory therapy. I was working at a small hospital in Phoenix – in the kitchen – and one of the therapists asked me, "Do you think you might want to train in my department?" And I thought, *Well, yeah, anything to get me out of this hot kitchen.*

So I did that, and worked as an RT from 1977 until I decided to go back to school for my master's. I did some counseling for a while, and I liked it, but I always felt there was more for me somewhere else in health care. Once my son finished college and I knew I had him well on his way, I thought, *Well, maybe I'm going to explore going back to school to be a nurse.*

That young father's tumors were way too deep to remove. Right after diagnosis, he had undergone surgery, suffered through chemo, and finally had radiation treatments. Unfortunately, when they radiated that area, they had burnt the tissues, and the tumors were just coming through everywhere. Those were some of the most violent tumors I had ever seen, and I wanted to try some wound care. "Maybe I can do something to ease your discomfort," I told him. I knew I wasn't going to fix them. But he looked at me and said, "I can't tolerate that at all." I realized at that point he was close to the end. Even though my gut, as a nurse, said, *I really should do something about these*, I just had to realize that wasn't important. I had to make him comfortable and let him say goodbye to his kids.

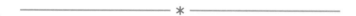

Back in my community college days, as part of an externship, I visited local hospitals and assisted social workers with some dying patients. That was when I first learned about hospice. The hospice movement had started in Europe many years earlier, but it wasn't until the early '70s that it started to reach the United States. Cecilia Saunders was one of the founders of hospice in England, and she had a profound influence on Elizabeth Kubler-Ross – the psychiatrist famous for her five-stages of-grief theory – who embraced hospice and holistic care at the end of life for comfort. Kubler-Ross lived her final years in Scottsdale, Arizona, and she was cared for by family and by nurses from the organization I work for now. So I did have that brief experience with hospice in the late '70s, and I loved it. But that was also the time I trained as a respiratory therapist, and I stayed with that for twenty-five years. I always knew that end of life work would be a special place for me to be, though. I just wasn't ready then to say, "Yup, I'll quit my job and head out."

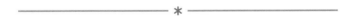

The second day I went back to that patient's house, he was in tears when he looked at me. "I'm in so much pain," he said. "I can't take it anymore. I'm not going to survive it this time." Up to that point, he had shown a surprisingly positive attitude. He had been saying, "I'm going to fight this. I can do it." But in that moment, he grabbed my hand, looked in my eyes, and said, "Bring my children to me, and my wife. I have to say goodbye to them because, after that, you're going to get me out of this pain."

I brought his family in. It just breaks me up to think about how he looked at his little seven-year-old and nine-year-old and told them how he was going with the angels, and how he was going to see them when they finally came to be angels themselves. He told them he would be there, and watch over them, and he'd always be with them. As soon as his wife and children went out, he looked at me again and said, "Do whatever you've got to do. I can't deal with this any longer."

I had my personal cell phone in one hand, and I was on my Blackberry in the other, trying to get orders to up his meds and get him comfortable. By the time he passed on Sunday evening, I had been able to actually stretch him out in his chair, so that his wife could see his face. He was a really handsome young man, and his wife was so grateful. She said, "Oh, my God, I haven't been able to see his face for the last three months without getting on the floor and looking up. I am just so thankful you made him comfortable enough that he could do it."

That was a tough one. But I say to myself, *You know what? We did it. We heard what he needed, we did what we needed to do, and we made his passing more peaceful and less traumatic for that whole family.*

The connection with hospice is at a very deep level for me. There has always been something saying to me that this is where I needed to be. And I'm a person who sort of follows my heart and my intuition a lot, and I knew a long time ago that eventually I would work in hospice. It just took me most of my life to get here, and I was still surprised by the way it happened.

In 2007, when I was still working as a respiratory program director, I was driving home from my office. I passed a sign for a job fair at Hospice of the Valley, and something mysterious inside me told me I needed to stop. I literally felt a call, almost on a spiritual level. I saw that sign out front and thought, *I'm just going to stop and see.* They interviewed me immediately and liked some of the skill sets I had, especially my background in respiratory therapy and my master's degree in counseling. Then they actually hired me right away, and I worked pool for them for a couple of years. Then, in 2009, they brought me on full time. In retrospect, it seems so predestined that I still find myself wondering, *What made me stop? Why did I pass that sign on that day? Why did I feel such spontaneous urgency?*

Hospice of the Valley is, I think, the largest hospice in the country, and they're incredibly passionate about caring for people. I've never worked in such a positive company. They really offer nurturing experiences, so it's easy to thrive in this environment. It's a big enough company that we have palliative home care, home health, and different inpatient units throughout Maricopa County, and I've had the opportunity to do a little bit of everything. I like variety in my life, and I enjoy knowing I can step into any role. Most of the time, though, I work in patients' homes. When someone is in crisis, we'll bring nurses in 24/7, stay there until we can get their symptoms under control, and train the family to be able to transition that care back.

My usual script is meant to explain what we do and offer some immediate structure that will counteract the despair and chaos we often find. I'll tell people, "We're part of a specialized crisis team, here to help manage the symptoms that you're feeling overwhelmed by right now. We'll stay here for a few days, until the situation is under control, and we'll teach you how to assist your loved one. After that, you won't be alone, because we have twenty-four-hour coverage with triage nurses. You can always pick up the phone and talk to somebody, and if it's something they can't rectify over the phone, they'll send another nurse out. Even if it's the middle of the night, we'll do what we need to do. We will be there for you, always, even though I may not be here in the home for twelve hours straight."

When I'm with patients and their families, I listen carefully to everything they say, and I try to decipher what their real needs are. I had a patient last year, and it truly was end of life for her – she died within a couple of weeks of us arriving at her home. She and her husband lived on a big property out in Cave Creek, Arizona, and she had horses. Before she died, she wanted to sit outside with this one particular horse. She had a tracheotomy tube in, so I dragged all the equipment outside with her and wheeled her underneath a tree. Her husband led her horse up, and she spent about half an hour out there, just petting her horse and talking to him. Watching her make that final connection and say goodbye was really something special for me.

I've had many patients who, at some point, like that young father, have looked at me and said, "I don't want to feel this anymore. Do whatever you need to do to get me out of pain." Then it's just communicating with physicians and getting the appropriate orders to get them to a place where they can pass in comfort. Relieving a patient's suffering is an essential priority in hospice, but I also want to ensure that the families don't have to witness their loved ones screaming in pain, either. The memory of those final moments lasts forever, so I try hard to balance all the wants and needs and then do everything I can to create the most peaceful death. We don't euthanize people. I think sometimes people might think, *Oh, my God, you just give them so much medication that they die*. We give them the medication that is required to get them out of pain. If that's what they want, and they make that desire clear to me, then I'll do my best to make it happen.

It's often the little things in nursing that count the most. Providing a small comfort, like giving a patient a bath at the end of life, can make a huge difference. I once gave a facial to a young lady who was dying of cancer. She was one of those women who went online and bought all of these facial products. I asked her son to bring out all her boxes of special creams, and I said to her, "Tell me which ones you love the most, because I'm going to give you a facial." I massaged her face and her neck and rubbed in some different creams, and she said, "That was so wonderful. I couldn't have paid a hundred bucks and gotten a better one." And twenty-four hours later, she just peacefully went. Afterwards, her son said to me, "Boy, I know how much she enjoyed that."

There have been a couple of patients where I had to go home and just ask God, "Why? Why?" But then, my own belief system dictates that what happens to us on this earth is simply the result of unfortunate circumstances. I don't believe that God runs around giving people cancer so they can die a painful death. I just don't want to believe that. But there have been some young people that I've had to deal with, that I've seen die, where I thought, *This is just so sad to see somebody die like this, and to see the family so torn up and losing their child before he was ever able to marry or have children or anything.* As terrible as those situations were, though, my reactions have never made me feel I couldn't do this work anymore.

You should never give up on your true desires. If you want to do something, don't ever say to yourself, "I'm too old. I'll never get it. Why should I try now?" Like I said, in 2003 I was in my early fifties when I started the program to become a nurse. At that time, I really wasn't sure that I'd be able to finish it, even physically, because I was still working fifty hours a week as a program director. But once I got myself a calendar and I sat down and I thought, *You're going to do this, so just figure out the best way*, I got into the groove of it. Then, once I started earning As on all my exams, I felt like, *Wow, I guess I really can do this*. And it's funny, but there are still things I come across in nursing where I'll say, "I remember when I learned this. I remember that unit where they taught me this."

Maturity can come along with age, too, and I try to bring a kind of emotional and spiritual component to patient care that a lot of younger nurses may not offer. That's a big help for people who are dying. This really is where I am best fitted – at end of life, with patients, with families – where I know that I can make that transition for them more comfortable, and I can help that family understand their loss better. That's why I really love it, and I don't see myself ever leaving hospice work.

MICHAEL YANNOTTA

Why I became a nurse is simple: my family. As a journeyman toolmaker at thirty-three, I had a good job, but that job was outsourced to China. I had one child and another on the way, so I worked nights in a factory while I went to school, first, to become an LPN and then an RN. I've had quite a wild ride in this profession, and I am currently director of nursing services at a busy long-term care and skilled-nursing center. It's amazing how much you can learn from those who have such a hard time remembering anything.

At thirty-three, I decided to switch careers. I was working as a tool and die maker, which had traditionally been a good job. But unfortunately, we kept seeing more slowdowns, more layoffs, and hour cuts. I used to get sixty to seventy hours a week when I was twenty-five, with all the overtime I could handle. But by the time I turned thirty, I could barely get a full week's work.

I worked at companies in New Jersey as a journeyman toolmaker. I knew how to run a surface grinder, a lathe, a milling machine, an electrical discharge machine, and all the other machines in the machine shop. I would take some blueprints and raw metals, and I would convert them into plastic injection molds – a million and one products you use every day, from hand-wipes container lids to fish-tank filters. My own particular area of expertise was actually finishing. I could take any piece of metal and make it shine until it acted like a mirror. When the planes hit the towers, I was polishing a coat hanger. To this day, I have a piece of that coat hanger in my toolbox downstairs, and it's still shiny.

My daughter was born in 2002 at St. Peter's Hospital in New Brunswick, and in the process, we got a great education from the nurses. Before that, honestly, I didn't know what nurses did day to day. As I watched them, though, I became intrigued by the profession. I realized not only how many different things they had to do, but the other thought that went through my mind was, *How are you going to send this to China? How are you going to outsource this? You can't. This is something that I can take care of my family doing.*

So I found an LPN program at one of the county schools that was one year long, and I found a night job. I went to college from seven in the morning until four in the afternoon. Then I'd hurry from school straight to my job, and work from about 4:30 until midnight, which wasn't easy. But I got my LPN in 2004, and within a week of graduating, I had a job at Hartwyck at Oak Tree, one of the nursing homes here in New Jersey. I worked on a brain-trauma unit, and I made more money in my first year of nursing than I did in my last year as a tool maker. So the jump to nursing turned out just fine for me.

However, working on that brain-trauma unit was challenging. Most of the injuries were caused by drug overdoses or by car accidents. With drug overdoses, for instance, the hypoxia that causes the brain trauma can strand people between life and death: they're there, they're alive, they're reactive, but they can't communicate. They may be responsive in their minds, but we can't ever really be sure if they hear us. Sometimes they can blink.

Now there are others who aren't so severely injured and they are able to speak, but often they're completely inappropriate – screaming out randomly as if they had Tourette's syndrome – with no curb on their emotions. I mean, you want to talk about a sad situation: maybe it's your son who just had a terrible car accident, or maybe you didn't even know your daughter had a drug problem, but you came home and found her unresponsive on the couch – what a horrible thing, right? When they're eighteen, that's not what you want to see happen.

Most of my patients had tracheotomies and feeding tubes. They couldn't tell me what was bothering them, so I had to learn how to judge what was going wrong inside them. Now mind you, their brain is injured, so everything is wrong, and I was constantly forced to assess from the baseline of what their conditions had been an hour earlier. You have to make judgments based on what they look like and sound like – what you can objectively observe – because there is no subjective information available.

I had one case where a young man had been severely injured at his engagement party. He and his fiancée lived in an apartment building, and he had fallen off the balcony. In the hospital, his fiancée was there every single evening, sitting by his side. She never wavered, never stopped coming to see him, for many months. At first, he couldn't communicate at all, but slowly he began to make his needs known, and then he regained his ability to speak. Finally, he learned to walk again, and he was on his way to recovery. Whether or not they did get married, I don't know. But I watched him leave for home with her. In 2005, HBO did a documentary on brain injury, and their story was part of that show.

What I really learned in that job, though, was something about trust, because I saw a lot of families stand vigil at bedsides. This was their little boy, or this was their daughter who had just gone out with her boyfriend for an evening, and all of a sudden something horrible had happened to them. They had no idea what was coming next. And so a lot of those families would stay right there at the bedside, never leaving, hoping for some small twitch that would signal recognition.

The day that I realized I was a pretty good nurse was when a family said, "Okay, Mike, you're here. We're going to go home for a couple of hours. We'll be back later." When they start to trust that you're going to take care of their loved one, that's how you know you're doing the right thing for those patients.

It was definitely the hardest job I've ever had in nursing. But it was also the best experience. All these years later, I still draw on things I learned there. Whenever I talk to people who are going to nursing school, I recommend that they work for a while in a place like that: "Spend six months there, at least, and get to understand how to deal with those unique patients," I tell them. "You're going to learn assessment. You're going to learn how to spot changes in condition. You're going to learn signs and symptoms. You're going to learn about trust. And after that job, everything else will feel easy."

I worked on that brain-trauma unit for about eight months, and then I took a job with a different nursing home. We received patients primarily from hospitals, and we provided nursing care along with oversight by a physician. We also offered rehabilitation – physical therapy, occupational therapy, speech therapy – and over 90 percent of the time we sent our patients back home.

As soon as I took that job, though, I realized that I didn't want to remain an LPN. I wanted to grow in my career, and to do that I had to become an RN. I didn't want to go back to a full-time nursing school where I was working all night and going to school all day. That was a once-in-a-lifetime experience that I didn't want to repeat, and one that I wouldn't wish on my worst enemy. So I found a distance learning school that complemented my working schedule. I enrolled in 2007 and graduated in 2011.

During my four years of online learning, I discovered that what I was reading and learning in every course helped me directly in my job. Becoming more knowledgeable improved my fluency with our physicians, and I began to move ahead even before I graduated. I was promoted to charge nurse and then to unit manager. It was simply a matter of taking what I was learning and applying it to what I was doing every day. I was surprised at how comfortable I became, sitting and talking with the families of patients. Whatever problem their loved ones had, I could discuss a variety of options for their care and rehabilitation. And as soon as I graduated, I became assistant director of nursing in one of that company's busiest skilled-nursing facilities.

A wonderful thing happened at that nursing home. We had one patient who was close to 100 years old, and she was actively dying. She was seriously ill and very debilitated. Her grandson was getting married in Florida, and she was truly too sick to make the flight there. Her family asked if they could bring the wedding to her, after he got married, and perform a second wedding for her in the nursing home, and I said, "Of course."

I managed the unit where she lived, and we made some special arrangements. First of all, we made sure that everything was extra clean, and then we had the activities department put up some ribbons to decorate the hallway. We moved around a few schedules so therapy sessions wouldn't get in the way, and we prepared the dining room so they could have a little reception in there.

They came in on a Friday, with the bride in her full makeup and wedding dress, and the groom, her grandson, who was actually in the

Marines, in his formal military uniform. They used our main hallway as the aisle. They also brought a reverend with them, along with all the bridesmaids and the groomsmen and the guests – a full wedding materialized there. Over the PA system, we played Pachelbel's Canon in G.

Well, that centenarian grandmother was just beaming. If you could have seen the look on that lady's face, it really spoke volumes. Remember, this was in a nursing home, so all of the patients could just come out of their rooms and see what was going on. Some were ambulatory, but others used their wheelchairs or walkers. Everybody came out and watched, and there wasn't a dry eye in the house. I don't think I'll ever see anything like that again. It's certainly something that touched my heart. Unfortunately, that lady passed away about a month later, but at least she died with that sweet memory. I would venture to bet that if we went back and checked the use of pain medication by our patients on the day of that wedding, we would see a measurable reduction. With the infectious joy that ran through that building, there's no way we wouldn't.

This has always been my philosophy about nursing homes: you're someplace where nobody wants to be, because if you had your choice, you'd go home. If you weren't sick, and if there wasn't something that was radically wrong, you'd be anyplace else in the world but there. So I take it as part of the job, part of our daily routine, to make life as enjoyable as we can. If that means that somebody needs to have her blinds closed because the sun annoys her, or if someone else has to be adjusted in his bed every two minutes, because that's what will make him a little more comfortable, then that's what we need to do. I feel like we just have to take that kind of caring approach.

Currently I am the director of nursing services at a busy long-term care and skilled-nursing facility, and most of the patients in my facility are in their seventies and eighties. They've lived their long lives taking care of themselves, for the most part. If they need some extra attention late in their lives, we shouldn't begrudge them. There's a common misconception that I try to dispel: many nurses will say, "I'm not your waitress. I'm not your maid." But at the end of the day, for our patients, I think our nurses and aides have to be their everything.

Our residents would do it for themselves if they could. They've had to give up independence and freedom, so we need to give them a break. If they want us to get them an extra glass of water, or another cookie, there's nothing wrong with that.

The only patients who really bother me are the ones who, for whatever reason, grow violent. Remember that dementia and Alzheimer's are a constant fact of life in nursing homes, and the patients who kick, bite, slap, spit, scream, or throw things at you on a daily basis seldom know what they're doing. Usually, in cases like that, it's not the patient who frustrates the nurse or the health care worker – it's the patient's family. The family may not see the behaviors or understand them when they do occur. They may not know that this person has dementia and they're acting out in this violent manner, because when they come by to pay a visit, the patient is often sleeping. Or the patient may have just finished dinner and they're postprandial and relaxed. But in the morning or late in the evening, those same patients might be running around, trying to hit everybody.

I had one fellow in particular who had been in the construction trades all his working life and, even in his eighties, was still very strong, with big, powerful arms. He was downright scary at times, and it was hard to curb his behaviors. It took about three or four months to get something figured out, and in the end, it was an accidental discovery. One day, when he was threatening a staff member, a nurse handed him a doll that looked like a baby. "Hey, the baby's sleeping. Can you hold him?" she asked. And he sat down with the doll, became very quiet, and just held onto it. Who would ever have thought that would work?

I've done a lot of things in my life. I drove tow trucks. I was a toolmaker. I worked in a restaurant. I did all kinds of different things as a young man, and I never had the satisfaction that I have now when I help somebody go home, or when I teach somebody for the first time how to take care of their diabetes. I know that for the rest of their lives they're going to remember what I did for them.

When all is said and done, if you want to talk about a job that comes with satisfaction that can't be measured, this is it. There will never be a paycheck that covers what I do in a day. There will never be a value placed on the services I provide. But at the end of the day, I also understand that some families of the people that I'm helping don't appreciate it one bit and are actually angry because their loved one is sick, or has gone downhill and is dying. They'll never realize what it is we do or why we do it.

However, watching somebody go from completely brain-injured to walking and talking again, or seeing somebody who has had his life shattered by a stroke get better and be able to go home – those are priceless experiences. I can give that stroke victim a hug and say, "Hey, good luck to you. Give me a call in a week and let me know how you're doing." And when they actually call me and say they're still doing okay, there's no greater job satisfaction than that.

AFTERWORD

It is with much gratitude that I thank the author, Bill Patrick, and the talented staff of Hudson Whitman/Excelsior College Press, led by Susan Petrie, for their work in making these moving stories known to us. The result is a rare opportunity to understand the various complexities of deciding to "heed the call" and become a nurse. Money, prestige, and attractive working conditions do not appear to be primary motives for the nurses in this book. What does emerge clearly is the shared desire to make a profound difference in the lives of others. As Florence Nightingale once said, "Rather, ten times, die in the surf, heralding the way to a new world, than stand idly on the shore." Like Nightingale, these individuals have sought to be involved and to make a contribution – both to other individuals and to our society.

What also comes through in these life narratives are the barriers and hardships that these nurses had to overcome to achieve their career goals. While perhaps unintended, the rigidity of a process which sends an adolescent, high school graduate from the classroom to the wards of the sick and injured often denies opportunities to many who may be older, already working, or encumbered by family and community responsibilities.

The fact that each of the nurses profiled here earned at least one of their higher education degrees in nursing from Excelsior College (or "Regents" before the name change) is no accident. Ours is the only nursing program that has been specifically designed for *experienced* working adults who cannot give up work to become full-time students. It provides the flexibility of independent preparation for a battery of examinations and gives worth to those years of *clinical* experience gained on the job. Yet, *no one* graduates from this program without passing a multi-day, hands-on assessment of clinical competency conducted in an acute-care facility with real patients.

Excelsior's approach to nursing education has helped to reduce America's nursing shortage: we have graduated nearly 50,000 new nurses in the last forty years, and our nursing program has at one time or another been recognized and accepted by all fifty states. It has also been reviewed and approved by the State of New York, the Middle States Commission on Higher Education (Excelsior's regional accreditor), the National League of Nursing's Accrediting Commission (since 1975), and has been named a "Center of Excellence in Nursing Education" continuously since such a designation was created by the NLN.

Excelsior College is proud of all of its graduates. We are especially proud of our nursing graduates who, as the earlier quote reminds us, continue to fight "the surf" (of restrictive models of nursing education) in order to show us "a new world" (one where experience is recognized and assessed for its true value).

Last, but by no means least, we offer thanks to those profiled here. Your openness and trust in sharing your experiences in health care are greatly appreciated. I am also gratified that you chose Excelsior (Regents) and its School of Nursing to assist you onto the path of becoming an RN. You represent the best in nursing, and you give credence to a model of preparation that we hope will "herald the way to a new world" in which the invaluable contributions of all nurses are finally recognized.

John Ebersole
President of Excelsior College

ACKNOWLEDGMENTS

I want to thank the nurses who volunteered for this project, and I'd like to explain why. This kind of book demands a lot of its participants. Of the 140 nurses who responded to an initial e-mail that asked for people who were willing to talk about their careers in health care, I chose fifty-seven. I conducted lengthy phone interviews with each of them and asked difficult questions, some of which tugged pretty hard at the corners of the HIPAA envelope or pried into personal areas that made some people uncomfortable. Forty-six nurses survived that round.

Once all forty-six interviews were transcribed into about 1800 pages of text, I sent those transcriptions out to the nurse-participants so they could see what they had explained and confessed in the heat of the interview process. The reality of a conversation converted to print, especially in the unvarnished form of an interview transcription that can't reveal inflection or nonverbal emotion, proved unnerving for a few more. And at that point, when I also asked the remaining nurses to sign a legal permission form that granted Hudson Whitman/Excelsior College Press publication rights for their stories and photographs, the field narrowed to forty.

The final step in the process involved transforming the transcriptions into readable stories. That meant I had to create dramatic monologues that presented a variety of coherent narrative structures that don't exist in regular conversation, or in interview transcriptions. When people tell you about what they've experienced in their lives, they don't formulate abstractions – they tell stories. So I did my best to retain the actual, colloquial words spoken by each nurse, only deviating to avoid repetitions or to clarify points. And I certainly didn't want to invent anything, because responsible nonfiction is one of the few remaining refuges of authenticity.

When I e-mailed the stories I had written to the nurses for their final review, several more backed out or wanted to change the most revealing parts so they wouldn't get into trouble at their jobs. I sympathized with their apprehensions, but that self-censorship still reduced my story pool to thirty-six. In the end, because the material was so rich, the stories ran longer than I had estimated at the beginning of the project, and the realities of publishing dictated that I could only include twenty-three.

None of these nurses was paid a dime for what they contributed to this project, and there would be no book without their selfless generosity. And there would definitely be no book worth reading without their willingness to share the most compelling aspects and experiences of their careers. This is more than a book of health care stories, and far more than just excerpts from random conversations with people who are describing their specific occupational trenches. This is an anthology of hard-won wisdom, and I celebrate the courage of these nurses for offering their version of it.

WILLIAM B. PATRICK

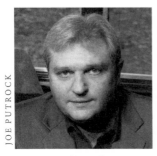

JOE PUTROCK

William B. Patrick is a writer whose works have been published or produced in several genres: creative nonfiction, fiction, screenwriting, poetry, and drama. His most recent book, *Courageous Learning: Finding a New Path through Higher Education*, appeared in October 2011 from Hudson Whitman/Excelsior College Press.

Saving Troy, his innovative chronicle of a year spent riding with professional firefighters and paramedics, was published in 2005. From that experience, Mr. Patrick also wrote a screenplay, *Fire Ground*, as well as a radio play, *Rescue*, which was commissioned by the BBC for its Season of American Thirty Minute Plays and which aired on BBC 3.

His memoir in poetry, *We Didn't Come Here for This*, was published by BOA Editions. In a starred review, *Kirkus* called the book a "marvelous memoir-in-poetry and a wonderful hybrid, written in a voice that's compassionate, fresh and American, without ever proclaiming itself such."

Mr. Patrick's novel, *Roxa: Voices of the Culver Family*, won the 1990 Great Lakes Colleges Association New Writers Award for the best first work of fiction.

ABOUT HUDSON WHITMAN

Hudson Whitman is a new, small press affiliated with Excelsior College in upstate New York.

Our tagline is "Books That Make a Difference," and we aim to publish high-quality nonfiction books and multimedia projects in areas that complement Excelsior's academic strengths: education, nursing, health care, military interests, business & technology, with one "open" category, American culture & society.

If you would like to submit a manuscript or proposal, please review the guidelines on our website, hudsonwhitman.com. Feel free to send a note with any questions. We endeavor to respond as soon as possible.

OTHER TITLES BY HUDSON WHITMAN

Shot: Staying Alive with Diabetes
Amy F. Ryan (print and e-book)

The Language of Men: A Memoir
Anthony D'Aries (print and e-book)

Courageous Learning: Finding a New Path through Higher Education
John Ebersole and William Patrick (print and e-book)

Saving Troy: A Year with Firefighters and Paramedics in a Battered City
William Patrick (e-book only)